MCQ Companion to the
Textbook of Anaesthesia

This book is due for return on or before the last date shown below.

For Churchill Livingstone

Publisher Michael Parkinson
Project Editor Jane Shanks
Project Controller Frances Affleck
Copy Editor Alison Gale
Design Direction Erik Bigland

MCQ Companion to the Textbook of Anaesthesia

David Fell
MB ChB FRCA
Consultant Anaesthetist
Leicester Royal Infirmary,
Leicester, UK

David Derbyshire
MB ChB FRCA
Consultant Anaesthetist,
Warwick General Hospital,
Warwick, UK

Graham Smith
BSc MD FRCA
Professor of Anaesthesia,
University of Leicester,
Leicester, UK

Alan Aitkenhead
BSc MD FRCA
Professor of Anaesthesia,
University Hospital,
Queens Medical Centre,
Nottingham, UK

SECOND EDITION

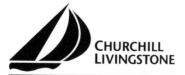

CHURCHILL
LIVINGSTONE

EDINBURGH LONDON NEW YORK PHILADELPHIA SYDNEY TORONTO 1998

CHURCHILL LIVINGSTONE
An imprint of Harcourt Brace & Company Limited

Robert Stevenson House, 1–3 Baxter's Place,
Leith Walk, Edinburgh EH1 3AF, UK

First published 1998

ISBN 0 443 05346 4

British Library of Cataloguing in Publication Data
A catalogue record for this book is available from the British Library.

Library of Congress Cataloging in Publication Data
A catalog record for this book is available from the Library of Congress.

Medical knowledge is constantly changing. As information becomes
available, changes in treatment, procedures, equipment and the use of
drugs become necessary. The author and publisher have, as far as it is
possible, taken care to ensure that the information given in the text is
accurate and up to date. However, readers are strongly advised to
confirm that the information, especially with regard to drug usage,
complies with current legislation and standards of practice.

Produced by Addison Wesley Longman China Limited, Hong Kong
EPC/01

Preface

Since the first edition of this book was published in 1991, the FRCA has reverted to a two-part examination. The Primary examination combines the assessment of knowledge of basic sciences and clinical anaesthesia. The written answers which formed part of the old Part 1 examination have been abolished. The examination now comprises multiple choice questions (MCQs), an objective structured clinical examination (OSCE) and two oral examinations, one of which is devoted to basic science topics. Candidates who fail the MCQ section in all its aspects are not permitted to proceed to the OSCE and oral examinations. Thus, appropriate preparation for the MCQ examination is essential.

The main aims of this book are to act as a companion to *Textbook of Anaesthesia*, third edition, edited by A. R. Aitkenhead and G. Smith, and to provide a set of questions and answers which we hope will help candidates to practise their technique of answering MCQs and to assess their progress in the acquisition of a sufficient depth of knowledge to approach the Primary FRCA examination with confidence.

The encouraging responses to the three editions of *Textbook of Anaesthesia* suggest that the book has been useful, presenting material appropriate both to the new recruit into anaesthesia and during the first 2–3 years in the specialty. As the syllabus for the Primary FRCA examination is based on the knowledge expected of an anaesthetist at the latter stage of training, *Textbook of Anaesthesia* should also fulfil its aim of providing suitable material for the examination candidate. An MCQ book based on *Textbook of Anaesthesia* is therefore likely to reflect the standard expected of the Primary examination candidate.

In this second edition, the sections on physiology and pharmacology have been updated to include newer information and drug references. All the questions have been reviewed and, where necessary, revised, and new questions have been added. We believe that it is important to point candidates to sources of information in areas in which they have identified a gap in their knowledge, rather than simply present the answers with no explanation or with potentially confusing statements. Consequently we have cross-referenced the answers where appropriate with the relevant chapters in *Textbook of Anaesthesia*, third edition (1996). However, there are areas in which reference to *Textbook of Anaesthesia* is inappropriate and we have therefore included cross-references to a standard textbook of medicine, *Davidson's Principles and Practice of*

Medicine, 18th edition (1999) by C. Haslett et al., and to *British National Formulary*, Number 34 (September 1997).

It should be emphasized that this companion to *Textbook of Anaesthesia* is not intended to reproduce questions in the Primary FRCA bank of questions, and cannot be comprehensive in its coverage of potential examination topics. However, it is our hope that the book will help candidates to read and prepare efficiently and effectively for the Primary FRCA examination, that it will provide practice in answering MCQs at an appropriate level, and above all, that it will stimulate interest in and the acquisition of knowledge about anaesthesia.

Leicester, Warwick and Nottingham, 1998.
D.F.
D.R.D.
A.R.A.
G.S.

Introduction

There are many MCQ tutors and primers which provide a means of educational self testing and practice for prospective examination candidates. Some books arrange MCQ questions under topic headings and others provide topics in random order. The latter system is similar to an actual examination with topics changing from question to question and in degree of difficulty. However, whilst this system mimics the examination, it may not be conducive to efficient learning, when candidates normally study textbooks systematically.

In this book, we have used both approaches. In the first four chapters we have classified topics into physiology, pharmacology, medicine and anaesthesia, each containing 100 questions. In addition, in the final two chapters we have provided mock test papers which consist of 60 questions on a mixture of subjects in order to mimic the format of an examination paper. In all chapters, we have arranged questions on the left side of the paper with answers and a brief explanation on the right to permit ease of checking; self testing may be undertaken by the simple expedient of covering the right-hand page whilst reading the question stems.

In the two test papers, the overall score should provide an indication of the reader's performance; although the pass marks vary from examination to examination, the reader should hope to achieve 40%, whilst 60% represents a very good mark.

The candidate should have a strategy for attempting MCQs in the examination. There are many texts which provide valuable advice and the following recommendations may be familiar. Each MCQ consists of a stem and five items or statements with a possible answer of 'true' or 'false'. In both the primary and final FRCA examination, the MCQs are marked with a positive mark for a correct response, whilst a mark is deducted for an incorrect response and zero is given where there is no response. Thus for each stem, the range of scores varies from –5 to +5. The negative marking system should not concern you unduly. The effect is the same as scoring +2 for correct, +1 for don't know and 0 for wrong; the only difference is the position of the pass mark! Clearly, it is most unwise to guess at an answer; if you do not know the answer, you should leave it blank. Some candidates in the past have assumed that, having answered some 60% of questions correctly, it is strategically appropriate to cease at that point. This is unwise. It is important to answer as many questions as possible about which you are confident. Read questions carefully, and in an actual examination take care when transferring your answers from the question paper to the computer marking sheet; it is a good idea to check each five or ten questions to ensure that your answers are not out of phase with the questions.

Practising MCQs is difficult for several reasons. Firstly, there is difficulty in finding 'examination equivalent' questions. Many trainees ask colleagues to remember questions from previous examinations and it is not unknown for departments to build up a stock of questions. However, the FRCA examination is reviewed continuously and the bank of questions enlarges and changes constantly. Secondly, there is difficulty in defining correct answers. There are only two allowable options, 'true' or 'false', but there is no provision for 'sometimes' which enters the thought processes of both examiners and candidates not infrequently! If this occurs to the candidate, we suggest that help may be forthcoming by considering the question in a different format. For example, if a question asks if a condition is associated with certain other processes, the candidate should ask himself if these processes are clinically important or unimportant – if not, the answer is more likely to be negative.

Throughout this text, we have been brief in our explanations because providing a full explanation might have resulted in a textbook in itself! By referencing one of only three readily available books, we trust that impetus will be given to readers to consolidate their knowledge from these texts.

Abbreviations

The following abbreviations are employed in the answer sections:

A & S   Aitkenhead A R, Smith G 1996 Textbook of Anaesthesia 3rd edn. Churchill Livingstone, Edinburgh (Ch indicates the relevant chapter number)

D   Edwards C R W, Bouchier I A D, Haslett C 1999 Davidson's Principles and Practice of Medicine 18th edn. Churchill Livingstone, Edinburgh (Ch indicates the relevant chapter number)

BNF   British National Formulary 34, 1997, British Medical Association and the Pharmaceutical Society (Ch indicates the relevant chapter number; Ch Em = Emergency Treatment of Poisoning).

DF
DRD

Contents

1. Physiology

1 Functional residual capacity (FRC)
a represents about 75% of vital capacity.
b may be measured by nitrogen washout.
c is increased in the elderly.
d is increased in the supine position.
e is always greater than closing volume.

2 Aldosterone acts to
a reduce Na⁺ absorption in the proximal convoluted tubule.

b reduce Na⁺ diffusion in the descending loop of Henle.

c increase Na⁺ absorption in the distal convoluted tubule.

d reduce Na⁺ absorption in the distal convoluted tubule.
e increase Na⁺ absorption in the collecting ducts.

3 Albumin
a has a molecular weight of approximately 70 000 daltons.
b has a plasma concentration of 35–50 g/l.

c concentration is increased in chronic liver disease.

d concentration is increased in malabsorption syndrome.
e is a major contributor to plasma oncotic pressure.

(Ch. 1, Appendix VIII, A & S)

a **False** Normally, FRC is less than 50% of vital capacity.
b **True** But helium dilution is used more commonly.
c **False** FRC decreases slightly with age.
d **False** FRC decreases when supine.
e **False** Closing volume may exceed FRC in the elderly and in the supine position.

(Ch. 3, A & S; Ch. 6, D)

a **False** Approximately two-thirds of the filtered sodium load is absorbed actively and passively in the proximal convoluted tubule; this is not influenced by aldosterone.
b **False** The descending limb of the loop of Henle is freely permeable to water, sodium and chloride and is not under the influence of aldosterone.
c **True** This is the main action of aldosterone. Excretion of potassium ions is increased.
d **False** See **c** above.
e **True** Sodium conservation occurs also in the collecting ducts in response to aldosterone.

(Ch. 3, A & S)

a **True**
b **True** Albumin comprises the major portion of plasma protein concentration (Appendix. IV, A & S).
c **False** The serum albumin concentration is low in chronic liver disease.
d **False** Hypoalbuminaemia is likely, and results in oedema.
e **True** Oncotic pressure in the normal individual represents the osmotic pressure of plasma proteins, of which albumin is the major part.

4 **The oxyhaemoglobin dissociation curve (ODC) is shifted to the left by**
  a acidosis.

  b nitric oxide.
  c hypercapnia.
  d decrease in temperature.
  e reduced concentration of 2,3-diphosphoglycerate (2,3-DPG).

5 **Normal atmospheric pressure is approximately**
  a 760 mmHg.
  b 1000 kPa.
  c 1000 cmH_2O.
  d 1000 millibar.
  e 14.7 lb. in^{-2}.

6 **Stroke volume**
  a is a determinant of cardiac output.
  b is unaffected by preload.

  c is related normally to afterload.

  d is determined normally by heart rate.

  e is independent of myocardial contractility.

7 **The following are endogenous CNS neurotransmitters:**
  a acetylcholine.

  b serotonin (5-HT).
  c magnesium.
  d GABA.
  e glutamate.

8 **Systemic arterial pressure is increased**
  a on assumption of the erect from the supine position.
  b on sudden exposure to cold.
  c always when heart rate increases.

  d by carotid sinus hypoxia.

  e in response to stimulation by peripheral chemoreceptors.

a **False** The ODC is shifted to the right by an increase in temperature, hydrogen ion concentration, carbon dioxide tension and 2,3-diphosphoglyceric acid concentration. Decreases in these variables cause a leftward shift of the ODC.
b **False**
c **False** See **a** above.
d **True** See **a** above.
e **True** See **a** above. 2,3-DPG concentration is reduced in stored blood.

---

a **True**
b **False** It is 101.3 kPa.
c **True**
d **True**
e **True**

---

a **True** Cardiac output = heart rate × stroke volume.
b **False** Stroke volume is proportional to preload. This is the Frank–Starling law.
c **False** But in the failing ventricle, stroke volume increases with decreasing afterload.
d **False** But at very high heart rates, there is decreased ventricular filling time and stroke volume may decrease.
e **False** There is a direct relationship.

---

a **True** Acetylcholine is in the motor nerves and CNS ascending pathways.
b **True** 5-HT occurs in the brain stem and spinal cord.
c **False**
d **True** GABA is the inhibitory neurotransmitter.
e **True** Glutamate is an excitatory neurotransmitter.

---

a **False** Arterial pressure tends to decrease initially.
b **True** Because of peripheral vasoconstriction.
c **False** This increases cardiac output, but does not necessarily influence systemic arterial pressure.
d **True** Systemic arterial pressure is increased in response to increased sympathetic activity, with chemoreceptor stimulation.
e **True** Stimulation of peripheral chemoreceptors mainly causes hyperventilation.

9   Carbon dioxide is transported in the blood mostly
   a   as carboxyhaemoglobin.

   b   in combination with plasma protein.

   c   as bicarbonate.

   d   dissolved in plasma as carbonic acid.

   e   at a partial pressure of 5.3 kPa in mixed venous blood.

---

10   Which statements are true of cranial nerves?
   a   The vagus supplies all the intrinsic muscles of the larynx.
   b   All intrinsic muscles of the tongue are supplied by the hypoglossal nerve.
   c   The abducent nerve supplies the lateral rectus muscle.
   d   The baroreceptors are innervated by the cranial root of the accessory nerve.
   e   The glossopharyngeal subserves sensation from the posterior third of the tongue and all of the epiglottis.

---

11   During pregnancy
   a   plasma fibrinogen concentration is increased.
   b   plasma cholinesterase concentration is increased.
   c   there is an increase in FRC.

   d   haemoglobin concentration is decreased.

   e   absorption of calcium ions via the gut is increased.

---

12   The neuromuscular junction
   a   has a junctional cleft of 60 nm.
   b   has muscarinic acetylcholine receptors on the postjunctional membrane.
   c   has a transmembrane potential of 90 mv at rest.
   d   is an example of a tight junction.
   e   has presynaptic acetylcholine receptors.

(Ch. 1, A & S)
a **False** Carboxyhaemoglobin is the compound formed by combination of carbon monoxide with haemoglobin.
b **False** Combination of carbon dioxide with plasma protein does not occur.
c **True** This involves ionization of carbonic acid and the Hamburger shift.
d **False** Carbonic acid dissociates into hydrogen ions and bicarbonate ions.
e **False** The partial pressure of carbon dioxide is about 6 kPa in mixed venous blood.

(Ch. 4, A & S; Ch 14, D)
a **True** Via the superior and recurrent laryngeal nerves.
b **True**

c **True**
d **False** Impulses from baroreceptors are carried in the carotid sinus nerve, a branch of the glossopharyngeal nerve.
e **False** The posterior part of the epiglottis is innervated by the vagus nerve.

(Ch. 5, A & S)
a **True** This occurs from the second trimester.
b **False** Plasma cholinesterase concentration is decreased by 30%.
c **False** FRC is decreased in pregnancy, as a result of a decrease in residual volume.
d **True** Plasma volume increases more than the increase in red cell mass, with a resultant decrease in haemoglobin concentration.
e **False** Absorption capacity for calcium is unchanged. The increased needs of pregnancy may result in calcium deficiency.

(Ch. 11, A & S)
a **True** The cleft contains acetylcholinesterase.
b **False** The acetylcholine receptors here are nicotinic.

c **True** The inside is negative.
d **False** These appear in the renal tubules.
e **True** This is part of the positive feedback mechanism.

13 **In comparison with intracellular fluid, extracellular fluid has**
a greater volume.

b greater potassium concentration.

c lower bicarbonate concentration.
d greater chloride concentration.
e greater osmolality.

14 **Gastric emptying**
a is delayed by anxiety.
b normally occurs exponentially.
c occurs in response to secretion of intrinsic factor.
d is controlled by duodenal osmoreceptors.
e is delayed in advanced pregnancy.

15 **Catecholamine release is stimulated by the following:**
a hypoxaemia.

b hypothermia.

c hypoglycaemia.

d hypercapnia.
e hypocalcaemia.

16 **Insulin causes**
a reduced gluconeogenesis.

b increased glycogenolysis.

c synthesis of proteins from amino acids.

d entry of potassium into cells.

e lipolysis.

(Ch. 3, A & S)

a **False** Total body water comprises approximately 60% of body weight; two-thirds of the water is intracellular.
b **False** Potassium forms the major intracellular cation, with a concentration of approximately 150 mmol/l.
c **False**
d **True** Chloride is present in cells in a concentration of only 10 mmol/l.
e **False** Osmolality is similar in extracellular and intracellular fluids.

(Ch. 31, A & S; Ch. 9, D)

a **True** And by pain and opioid analgesia.
b **True**
c **False** Intrinsic factor promotes vitamin B_{12} absorption.
d **True** Increased duodenal osmolality delays gastric emptying.
e **True** But returns to normal after delivery.

(Ch. 22, A & S)

a **True** The tachycardia associated with hypoxaemia is secondary to sympatho-adrenal activity.
b **False** Hypothermia reduces basal metabolic rate and catecholamine secretion.
c **True** Hypoglycaemia stimulates catecholamine release, producing the characteristic signs of sweating and tachycardia *(Ch. 8, D)*.
d **True** Carbon dioxide retention stimulates catecholamine release.
e **False** There is no effect of hypocalcaemia on the sympatho-adrenal axis.

(Ch. 8, D)

a **True** Insulin causes glucose uptake by the cell and inhibits gluconeogenesis.
b **False** Glycogenolysis is the breakdown of glycogen to starch and sugar. This is inhibited by insulin.
c **True** Insulin is an anabolic hormone. The absence of insulin leads to protein breakdown.
d **True** Reduced plasma concentrations of insulin lead to hyperkalaemia.
e **False** Lack of insulin leads to lipolysis.

17 Severing the cervical sympathetic trunk results in
a dilatation of the pupil.
b reduction in sweating.
c partial ptosis.

d decreased taste sensation on the anterior two-thirds of the tongue.
e dry oral mucous membrane.

18 The following occur postoperatively:
a increased secretion of antidiuretic hormone (ADH).

b increased loss of potassium.

c decreased loss of sodium.
d decreased urine osmolality.

e increased FRC.

19 Alveolar P_{CO_2} (P_{ACO_2})
a has a normal range of 4.8–5.8 kPa.
b differs from arterial P_{CO_2} by 1–1.5 kPa.
c is reduced by increased minute ventilation.
d is identical in value to mixed venous P_{CO_2}.
e is similar in value to end-tidal CO_2.

20 Gastrointestinal motility
a is inhibited by gastrin.
b is increased by vagal stimulation.
c is increased by sympathetic block.

d is increased by moderate distension.

e is diminished during labour.

(Ch. 14, D)

a **False** Pupillary constriction – miosis occurs.
b **True** Anhidrosis is part of Horner's syndrome.
c **True** The levator palpebrae superioris is innervated partly by the sympathetic system, in addition to the seventh cranial nerve.
d **False** Taste on the anterior two-thirds of the tongue is subserved by the lingual nerve – a branch of the mandibular nerve.
e **False** The secretomotor supply to the mucous membrane is parasympathetic in origin.

(Ch. 21, A & S)

a **True** Increased production of ADH occurs postoperatively as part of the normal endocrine response to stress.
b **True** Increased serum cortisol concentration caused by stress leads to retention of sodium and water, and loss of potassium ions.
c **True** See **b** above.
d **False** Because of sodium and water retention and the effect of ADH, urine osmolality postoperatively is greater than normal.
e **False** FRC is reduced intraoperatively because of increased activity of muscles of expiration and cranial displacement of the diaphragm. In addition, FRC may be reduced after abdominal or thoracic surgery because of pain and splinting of the diaphragm *(Ch. 1, A & S)*.

(Ch. 1, A & S)

a **True** This reflects arterial P_{CO_2} *(Appendix VIIIc, A & S)*.
b **False** See **d** below.
c **True** The relationship is hyperbolic.
d **False** Alveolar P_{CO_2} is equal to arterial P_{CO_2} in the normal patient.
e **True** End-tidal CO_2 approximates to alveolar P_{CO_2} in healthy lungs, but is lower in patients with increased $\dot{V}/\dot{Q}$ mismatch.

(Ch. 9, D)

a **False**
b **True**
c **True** Sympathetic block permits unopposed action of the parasympathetic nervous system *(Ch. 25, A & S)*.
d **True** Distension of the gut causes reflex stimulation of intestinal activity. However, activity is decreased in the presence of gross distension.
e **True** Gastrointestinal activity is diminished during pregnancy and labour *(Ch. 5, A & S)*.

21 In the kidney
   a   most sodium is absorbed in the proximal tubule.
   b   glucose is not excreted if the serum glucose concentration is normal.
   c   tubular cells secrete ammonia.

   d   acetazolamide acts on tubular production of HCO_3^-.

   e   aldosterone is secreted by the juxtaglomerular apparatus.

---

22 At the start of a forced expiration against a closed glottis there is
   a   increased intrathoracic pressure.

   b   increased systolic arterial pressure.

   c   increased heart rate.

   d   raised right ventricular output.

   e   decrease in left ventricular output.

---

23 Gastric emptying is accelerated by
   a   erect posture.
   b   low pH in the antrum.
   c   cholecystokinin.

   d   increased osmotic pressure of the duodenal contents.
   e   secretin.

---

24 In the heart
   a   the sinoatrial node is situated in the wall of the right atrium.

   b   the normal resting potential of cardiac muscle is –80 to –90 mV.

   c   the PR interval of the ECG represents the duration of atrial depolarization.
   d   the normal PR interval of the ECG is greater than 0.2 s.
   e   atrial conduction is slowed by a decrease in temperature.

(Ch. 3, A & S)

a	**True**	70% of sodium aborption occurs in the proximal tubule.
b	**True**	Provided that the renal threshold for glucose is normal, glycosuria does not occur unless hyperglycaemia is present.
c	**True**	Tubular secretion of ammonia facilitates hydrogen ion excretion and bicarbonate conservation.
d	**True**	Acetazolamide is a carbonic anhydrase inhibitor, which interferes with bicarbonate reabsorption.
e	**False**	The juxtaglomerular apparatus is responsible for renin production; the renin–angiotensin system is responsible for aldosterone secretion by the adrenal gland.

(Ch. 2, A & S)

a	**True**	The Valsalva manoeuvre produces increased intrathoracic pressure.
b	**True**	There is a transient increase in systolic arterial pressure due to increased ejection from the left ventricle.
c	**False**	There is an initial transient decrease in heart rate with the Valsalva manoeuvre.
d	**True**	There is an initial increase in right ventricular output, followed rapidly by a decrease as venous return into the thorax is impeded.
e	**False**	There is an initial increase in left ventricular output, followed rapidly by a decrease in overall cardiac output.

(Ch. 31, A & S; Ch. 9, D)

a	**True**	Assumption of the erect posture enhances gastric emptying.
b	**False**	
c	**False**	Cholecystokinin is secreted in response to duodenal stimulation and inhibits gastric emptying.
d	**False**	This is part of the enterogastric reflex.
e	**False**	Secretin is released in parallel with cholecystokinin.

(Ch. 2, A & S)

a	**True**	The sinoatrial node lies in the wall of the right atrium, close to the superior vena cava.
b	**True**	The resting membrane potential is determined by the relative concentrations of potassium, as described by the Nernst equation *(Ch. 4, A & S)*.
c	**False**	Atrial depolarization is represented by the P wave.
d	**False**	The normal PR interval is 0.12–0.20 s *(Appendix IIIa, A & S)*.
e	**True**	A decrease in temperature decreases cellular activity including depolarization.

25 **The following are true:**
   a Sodium is the main determinant of extracellular fluid (ECF) osmolality.
   b Hypernatraemia results in intracellular dehydration.

   c K^+ is the main determinant of intracellular osmolality.

   d Acidosis increases intracellular K^+.

   e The combination of a low ECF chloride and normal sodium concentration indicates respiratory alkalosis.

---

26 **Lung compliance**
   a is the reciprocal of airways resistance.

   b is expressed as cmH_2O/l.

   c exhibits hysteresis.
   d is increased in the presence of pulmonary oedema.

   e is unaffected by anaesthesia.

---

27 **CSF normally has a**
   a protein content of 200–400 mg/l.

   b P_{CO_2} higher than that of arterial blood.

   c specific gravity of 1040.
   d pressure of 100 mmH_2O.

   e volume of about 60 ml in an average adult.

---

28 **The following are true of fluid balance:**
   a The fluid requirement of a 15 kg child is approximately 3.5 ml/kg per hour.
   b Insensible daily loss for a 70 kg man in a normal environment is more than 1200 ml.
   c Obligatory daily urine production in a normal environment for a 70 kg man is more than 800 ml.

   d The total body water of infants and small children is approximately 80% of body weight.
   e Total body water of infants and small children is 80 ml/kg body weight.

(Ch. 21, A & S)

a **True** ECF osmolality is normally approximately 300 mosmol/kg; sodium accounts for approximately 145 mosmol/kg.
b **True** Water moves along an osmotic gradient from intracellular to extracellular compartments.
c **True** Intracellular potassium concentration is approximately 150 mmol/l.
d **False** In acidosis, there is a shift in potassium from the intracellular to the extracellular compartment.
e **False** Chronic respiratory acidosis may result in hypochloraemia, secondary to compensatory bicarbonate conservation.

(Ch. 1, A & S)

a **False** Units of compliance contain no time-base, in contrast to those of resistance.
b **False** It is expressed as change in volume/change in pressure (litre/kPa).
c **True** This is due to the presence of surfactant.
d **False** The lungs are less compliant (stiffer) if pulmonary oedema is present.
e **False** Compliance decreases during anaesthesia.

(Chs. 4 and 37, A & S)

a **True** Protein content is lower than that of plasma, but may be increased in conditions such as Guillain–Barré syndrome.
b **False** Carbon dioxide diffuses readily between CSF and blood, but is buffered less efficiently in CSF; thus, acute changes in P_{CO_2} produce large changes in CSF pH.
c **False** Specific gravity is approximately 1005.
d **True** In the horizontal position, the pressure range is normally 100–150 mmH$_2$O.
e **False** Volume is approximately 120 ml and the CSF undergoes rapid (4-hourly) turnover.

(Ch. 21, Appendix VIa, Appendix IXc, A & S)

a **True** This child requires 1000 ml + 50 × [15–10] ml/24 h = 52 ml/h.

b **False** In a temperate climate, up to 1 l of water daily may be lost in expired air and by evaporation.
c **False** Urine osmolality may reach a maximum of 1200–1400 mosmol/kg; with a normal diet, the minimum volume of urine required is about 500 ml *(Ch. 3, A & S)*.
d **True** This varies from 75–85% of body weight and exceeds the value for an adult.
e **False** This is the blood volume of infants and small children.

29 With respect to the circulation in a healthy adult

a the major proportion of blood volume is accommodated in the low-pressure venous circulation.

b a decrease of up to 15% of blood volume is compensated by an increase in vasomotor tone.

c a 10% decrease in blood volume results in a reduction in cardiac output.

d arterial pressure is not a good index of blood loss.

e CVP decreases in response to a 10% reduction in circulating blood volume.

---

30 With respect to renal physiology

a about 200 l of water are filtered daily through the glomeruli.

b sodium filtration through the glomeruli is about 30 000 mmol/24 h.

c glomerular filtration rate (GFR) is constant over a wide range of systolic arterial pressure.

d normally, 90% of glomerular filtrate is reabsorbed.

e normally, at least 98% of filtered sodium is reabsorbed by the proximal tubules.

---

31 A serum sodium concentration of 142 mmol/l and serum potassium concentration of 6.2 mmol/l are compatible with

a hypopituitarism.

b Addison's disease.

c persistent severe hypovolaemia.

d myxoedema.

e stored CPD blood.

(Ch. 31, A & S)

a **True** The veins contain approximately 80% of the blood volume
(Ch. 2, A & S).
b **True** However, when 20% of the intravascular volume is lost,
tachycardia and orthostatic hypotension develop.
c **False** Most healthy adults can cope with a 10% decrease in
intravascular volume with no change in cardiac output.
d **True** However, in the elderly and those with compromised
circulatory reflexes, there is less tolerance to small decreases
in blood volume.
e **False** However, with loss of intravascular volume in excess of 10%,
a decrease in CVP occurs.

(Ch. 3, A & S)

a **True** Water and substances of small molecular weight pass through
the glomerular capillary wall.
b **True** Sodium passes through the glomerular capillary wall. The normal
plasma sodium concentration (150 mmol/l) multiplied by the
filtration rate (200 l/24 h) gives a value of about 30 000 mmol.
c **True** Cortical autoregulation maintains GFR constant over the range
of arterial pressure 90–180 mmHg.
d **False** Normally, 99% of glomerular filtrate is reabsorbed by the renal
tubules.
e **False** Although at least 98% of filtered sodium is reabsorbed in the
kidney, the proximal tubule accounts for approximately 70%.

(Ch. 8, D)

a **False** Secretion of aldosterone is unaltered in hypopituitarism, and
therefore potassium excretion is not usually abnormal.
b **False** Hyponatraemia is normally a feature of Addison's disease.
c **True** In severe circulatory failure there is impairment of potassium
excretion by the kidney, and potassium may be released from
cells damaged by trauma.
d **False**
e **True** Hyperkalaemia occurs in stored blood. The serum potassium
concentration may increase to this value within a few days of
storage *(Ch. 6, A & S)*.

32 Aldosterone

  a is a polypeptide.

  b is synthesized in the zona glomerulosa of the adrenal cortex.

  c acts on the proximal tubule of the kidney.

  d increases urinary [K+].

  e decreases urinary pH.

---

33 ADH

  a decreases the permeability of the collecting ducts of the kidney.

  b acts via cyclic AMP.
  c is secreted in response to neural stimuli originating in the hypothalamus.
  d is secreted in response to hypovolaemia, even if plasma is hypotonic.
  e is a decapeptide.

---

34 The sodium–potassium pump at the cell membrane
  a requires ATP.

  b is inhibited by digoxin.

  c maintains a low intracellular chloride concentration.

  d is responsible for active transport of sodium ions into the cell.

  e is responsible for generation of action potentials.

(Ch. 3, A & S)

a	**False**	Aldosterone is a mineralocorticoid with a steroid structure *(Ch. 8, D)*.
b	**True**	The zona glomerulosa is the outermost layer of the adrenal cortex.
c	**False**	Aldosterone acts on the distal tubule, to cause retention of sodium and excretion of potassium.
d	**True**	Potassium and/or hydrogen ions are secreted into the tubule in exchange for reabsorbed sodium. Thus, urinary potassium and hydrogen ion secretion are enhanced.
e	**False**	Although aldosterone increases tubular secretion of hydrogen ions, these are buffered.

(Ch. 3, A & S)

a	**False**	ADH increases the permeability of the collecting ducts to water. Thus urine volume is decreased.
b	**True**	Cyclic AMP acts as a second messenger.
c	**True**	Osmoreceptors in the hypothalamus detect changes in plasma osmolality.
d	**True**	ADH is part of the endocrine response to stress, and this overrides osmolar regulation.
e	**False**	It is an octapeptide, known also as 8-arginine vasopressin.

(Ch. 4, A & S)

a	**True**	Ion movement across the cell membrane occurs against an electrochemical gradient and therefore requires energy.
b	**True**	Cardiac glycosides increase the concentration of intracellular calcium by inhibition of sodium–potassium exchange at the cell membrane *(Ch. 13, A & S)*.
c	**False**	The cell membrane is permeable to chloride, which diffuses along an electrochemical gradient from intracellular to extracellular fluid.
d	**False**	Sodium is transported from inside to outside the cell against its concentration gradient.
e	**False**	The sodium–potassium pump is responsible for maintenance of the resting membrane potential and for repolarizing the membrane after depolarization by an action potential.

35 Renal blood flow

a   is subject to autoregulation.

b   is greater in the renal cortex than in the medulla.

c   may be measured using the Fick principle.

d   is approximately 10% of cardiac output.

e   is unaltered by haemorrhagic shock.

36 Active transport is involved in transfer across renal cell membranes of

a   potassium ions.

b   sodium ions.

c   glucose.

d   amino acids.

e   protein.

37 Which of the following are consistent with acute renal tubular necrosis?

a   oliguria.
b   a normal cortical blood flow.
c   increased urine urea concentration.

d   hyperkalaemia.

e   oedema.

(Ch. 3, A & S)

a **True** Autoregulation maintains constant renal blood flow in the face of changing perfusion pressure (within limits).

b **True** Autoregulation occurs in the cortex but not in the medulla. The afferent arteriole dilates when arterial pressure is decreased.

c **True** The Fick principle states that uptake or clearance of a substance by an organ is equal to its arteriovenous content difference multiplied by blood flow through the organ. In this case, *para*-aminohippuric acid (PAH) is used as the tracer substance.

d **False** The blood flow to the kidney is approximately 25% of cardiac output.

e **False** In haemorrhagic shock, medullary perfusion is impaired and, if blood pressure decreases below the lower limit of autoregulation, cortical perfusion is reduced also.

(Ch. 3, A & S)

a **True** Active sodium–potassium exchange occurs in the distal tubule and collecting duct.

b **True** In addition to **a** above, sodium is reabsorbed actively in the proximal tubule.

c **True** Almost 100% of glucose is reabsorbed by the proximal tubule unless Tm_g is exceeded.

d **True** Amino acids are transported actively out of the tubular lumen in the proximal tubule.

e **False** Protein does not appear in the glomerular filtrate under normal circumstances.

(Ch. 6, D)

a **True** Oliguria is a feature of acute tubular necrosis.

b **False** There is reduction in blood flow to the cortex.

c **False** Urinary urea concentration is decreased because of reduced GFR and impaired tubular function.

d **True** There is impaired ability to excrete potassium, and hyperkalaemia may require treatment with intravenous insulin and glucose.

e **True** Pulmonary oedema is a serious complication and may be caused by excessive administration of intravenous fluids.

38 A serum osmolality of 360 mosmol/kg is compatible with

a excessive secretion of ADH.

b normal serum.

c uraemia.

d freshwater drowning.

e uncontrolled diabetes mellitus.

39 Inulin

a is cleared completely from blood in a single passage through the kidney.

b is not reabsorbed from glomerular filtrate.

c is present in glomerular filtrate in a concentration equal to that in plasma.

d is secreted by the renal tubules.

e does not pass into the extravascular space.

40 Soluble insulin

a increases the entry of glucose into muscle cells.

b induces protein catabolism.

c increases the transport of amino acids into cells.

d is a polypeptide secreted by the alpha cells of the islets of Langerhans.

e has a duration of action of 12 h when given by subcutaneous injection.

(Ch. 3, A & S)

a **False** Excessive secretion of ADH results in water retention and a decrease in serum osmolality.
b **False** Normal serum osmolality is 280–300 mosmol/kg *(Appx. IV, A & S)*.
c **True** Urea contributes to serum osmolality.
d **False** Absorption of inhaled water is likely to lead to reduction in concentration of plasma constituents.
e **True** Hyperosmolar non-ketotic coma may occur, especially in the elderly diabetic *(Ch. 8, D)*.

(Ch. 3, A & S)

a **True** Inulin clearance represents GFR.

b **True** Because it is not reabsorbed from glomerular filtrate, its clearance represents GFR.

c **True** Because inulin is cleared in a single passage through the glomerulus, the concentration in the glomerular filtrate is equal to that in plasma. It should be noted that inulin has to be infused i.v. to achieve a steady plasma concentration.

d **False** It is neither absorbed nor secreted by the kidney tubules.
e **False** Inulin is a polymer with molecular weight 5000, and passes readily through capillary membranes into the extravascular space.

(Ch. 8, D)

a **True** This is the prime action of this endocrine hormone.
b **False** Insulin is an anabolic hormone which stimulates fat and protein synthesis. During the catabolic (stress) response to trauma and surgery, secretion of insulin is suppressed.
c **False** Insulin facilitates the entry of glucose, but not amino acids, into cells.
d **False** Insulin is a polypeptide which is secreted by the beta cells of the islets of Langerhans.
e **False** The duration of action of soluble insulin is approximately 6 h.

41 Cardiac muscle differs from skeletal muscle in that it
a has a longer refractory period.

b depolarizes spontaneously.

c can metabolize lactic acid.

d can only contract isometrically.

e has a low extraction ratio for oxygen.

42 Haemoglobin
a is a mucopolysaccharide.
b binds four molecules of oxygen per molecule.

c has a theoretical oxygen carrying capacity of 1.34 ml O_2/g.

d is catabolized in the reticuloendothelial system (RES).

e is an important buffer in the blood.

43 Cardiac output may be measured using
a PAH
b inulin.
c glucose.
d Evans blue.
e creatinine.

(Ch. 2, A & S)

a **True** Because of calcium influx, the period of depolarization (and therefore the refractory period) is prolonged.

b **True** The phase zero prepotential of cardiac muscle reflects leakage of sodium ions into the cell and a decrease in the leakage of potassium ions out of the cell. At a potential of –50 mV, spontaneous depolarization occurs.

c **False** Lactic acid may be produced in a hypoxic environment, but is not metabolized.

d **False** There is an isotonic phase of contraction as well as an isometric phase.

e **False** The extraction ratio of cardiac muscle is very high. The blood returning into the coronary sinus is amongst the most desaturated found in the body. Coronary venous P_{O_2} is approximately 4 kPa.

(Ch. 11, D; Ch. 1, A & S)

a **False** Haemoglobin is a protein.

b **True** The affinity of each haem fraction for each molecule of oxygen varies with the occupation of the other oxygen-carrying sites. It is this characteristic of haemoglobin which facilitates oxygen uptake and which results in the sigmoid oxyhaemoglobin dissociation curve.

c **False** The theoretical oxygen-carrying capacity of haemoglobin (Hufner's constant) is 1.39 ml/g, but the experimental value is 1.34 ml/g.

d **True** The principal catabolic site of haemoglobin is the monocyte–macrophage system (formerly RES) of the liver and spleen.

e **True** This is the Haldane effect.

(Chs. 2 and 3, A & S)

a **False** PAH is one of the substances used to measure renal plasma flow.

b **False** Inulin is used to measure glomerular filtration rate.

c **True** Cold glucose is part of the thermal technique.

d **True** Evans blue may be used for a dye dilution technique.

e **False** Creatinine is used to measure glomerular filtration rate.

44 The P_{50}

 a is increased by violent exercise.

 b is increased when blood pH decreases.

 c is unaffected by the operation of the Bohr effect.

 d is increased by increase in 2,3-DPG concentration in the erythrocytes.

 e is increased during ascent to high altitudes.

---

45 The Frank–Starling mechanism

 a relates force of contraction to fibre length.

 b does not operate in the human heart.

 c operates only in the denervated heart.

 d is abolished by changes in contractility.

 e is unaffected by afterload.

---

46 Cardiac output

 a may increase to values of 35 l/min during exercise.

 b is increased by vagal stimulation.

 c is uninfluenced by infusion of noradrenaline.

 d is increased by administration of adrenaline.

 e is increased when contractility increases.

(Ch. 1, A & S)

a **True** Violent exercise causes an increase in body temperature and this shifts the oxyhaemoglobin dissociation curve (ODC) to the right, causing an increase in the P_{50}.

b **True** This shifts the ODC to the right.

c **False** The Bohr effect is a shift to the right with increasing hydrogen ion concentration.

d **True** 2,3-DPG is produced by glycolysis; this shifts the ODC to the right, thus increasing the P_{50}.

e **False** Ascent to high altitude induces acute hyperventilation, with a decrease in P_{CO_2} and a consequent shift of the ODC to the left.

(Ch. 2, A & S)

a **True** The Frank–Starling mechanism states that force of contraction is determined by the initial fibre length.

b **False** Although originally described in animals, the principle may be applied in humans. Indirect indices of fibre length (e.g. LVEDP – left ventricular end-diastolic pressure) are used.

c **False** The mechanism operates in the denervated heart and also under normal circumstances.

d **False** Changes in contractility merely move the position of the curve relating contractility to initial fibre length.

e **False** Afterload affects LVEDP, and therefore initial fibre length.

(Ch. 2, A & S)

a **True** This occurs predominantly because of an increase in stroke volume.

b **False** Increased vagal tone decreases heart rate and, to a certain extent, contractility.

c **False** Noradrenaline increases afterload, causing decreases in heart rate and cardiac output. However, it may also exert an agonist action at beta-receptors, and in some circumstances increase cardiac output.

d **True** Adrenaline has positive inotropic and chronotropic actions.

e **True** Cardiac output depends upon heart rate and stroke volume. Stroke volume is increased with increasing contractility.

47 Pulmonary blood flow
a is distributed equally throughout the lung.

b is decreased by sympathetic stimulation.

c is unchanged during exercise.

d is uninfluenced by changes in alveolar P_{O_2}.

e is abnormal in the presence of significant pulmonary embolus.

---

48 In an ECG trace
a the paper speed is normally 2.5 cm/s.
b the PR interval is measured from the peak of the P wave to the peak of the R wave.
c the T wave becomes more peaked as the serum K^+ concentration increases.
d left ventricular hypertrophy is present when R in V_5 or V_6 plus S in V_1 is greater than 40 mm (4 mV).
e P waves are absent in atrial flutter.

---

49 The following are true for a blood sample with a P_{O_2} of 6.0 kPa:
a It is arterial blood; mean $\dot{V}/\dot{Q}$ ratio is less than normal.

b It is venous blood from a normal patient.
c Oxygen saturation is 80% (assuming normal pH, temperature, base excess, adult blood).
d It is 90% saturated fetal blood.

e It may be arterial blood from a patient with 50% right-to-left shunt.

a **False** 60% of right ventricular output is distributed to the lower 40% of lung volume in the erect position, because of the influence of gravity.
b **False** Sympathetic stimulation increases cardiac output and pulmonary blood flow.
c **False** Exercise-induced increases in cardiac output result in an increase in pulmonary blood flow.
d **False** A decrease in alveolar P_{O_2} causes hypoxic pulmonary vasoconstriction (HPV). This reflex is attenuated by inhalational anaesthetics (Ch. 38, A & S).
e **True** The greater the size of an embolus, the greater proportion of the pulmonary circulation is occluded.

(Ch. 3, D)

a **True** This is the conventional speed for ECG recording.
b **False** The PR interval is measured from the beginning of the P wave to the beginning of the R wave.
c **True** Tall, tented T waves are characteristic of hyperkalaemia (Ch. 5, D).
d **True**

e **True** P waves represent atrial depolarization in sinus rhythm. Flutter waves are present in the condition of atrial flutter.

(Ch. 1, A & S)

a **True** This represents severe hypoxaemia, which could be accounted for by a $\dot{V}/\dot{Q}$ ratio less than unity.
b **True** Normal mixed venous P_{O_2} is 6 kPa (Ch. 2, A & S).
c **True** Assuming a normal P_{50}, this would represent an oxygen saturation of 80%.
d **True** The oxyhaemoglobin dissociation curve of fetal haemoglobin has a lower P_{50} than that of adult haemoglobin, and a P_{O_2} of 6 kPa represents saturation of about 90% (Ch. 33, A & S).
e **True** A 50% shunt would result in a saturation of 80–85%, which corresponds to a P_{O_2} of 6 kPa, assuming a normal ODC.

50 FRC

a is the sum of the residual volume and the inspiratory reserve volume.

b is uninfluenced by posture.

c becomes less than closing volume with advancing age.

d is a measure of the resting expiratory position.

e may be measured by the helium dilution method.

51 The following variables are employed in Bohr's dead space equation:

a inspired P_{CO_2}.
b mean expired CO_2 concentration.
c Pc'_{CO_2}.
d tidal volume.
e cardiac output.

52 Peripheral chemoreceptors

a are in the carotid body.
b respond to carbon dioxide.
c respond to blood flow.
d control ventilation linearly in response to Sa_{O_2}.

e respond to a decrease in Hb concentration.

53 In a spontaneously breathing patient with upper respiratory obstruction, helium is beneficial because

a it is the best means of improving oxygenation.
b CO_2 elimination is achieved more easily.

c its viscosity overcomes small airways obstruction.
d its density overcomes large airways obstruction.

e it overcomes resistance in areas of laminar flow.

(Ch. 1, A & S)

a **False** FRC is the sum of the residual volume and expiratory reserve volume; it represents the volume in the lungs at the end of a normal tidal breath *(Appendix VIII, A & S)*.

b **False** FRC is reduced in the supine position.

c **True** Closing volume increases with increasing age and exceeds FRC in the elderly.

d **True** FRC represents a balance between the elastic recoil of the lungs and that of the chest wall at the end of expiration.

e **True** This is the standard method for measurement of FRC.

(Ch. 1, A & S)

a **False** Inspired CO_2 is usually negligible and is commonly ignored.

b **True**

c **False**

d **True**

e **False**

(Ch. 1, A & S)

a **True** They lie in the carotid and aortic bodies.

b **False** The central chemoreceptors respond to CO_2.

c **True**

d **True** The pulmonary ventilatory response to Sa_{O_2} is linear, but it is exponential to Pa_{O_2}.

e **False**

(Ch. 15, A & S)

a **False** The best way to improve oxygenation is to increase $F_{I_{O_2}}$.

b **True** A helium/oxygen mixture improves alveolar ventilation and may delay the onset of hypercapnic respiratory failure.

c **False** The viscosity of helium is similar to that of oxygen.

d **True** The lower density of helium compared with air or oxygen results in lower resistance in an obstructed upper airway, in which flow is turbulent.

e **False** Laminar flow depends upon gas viscosity, not density.

54 **An area in the lung with increased ventilation/perfusion ratio**
a represents shunt.
b represents dead space.
c is responsible for a decrease in Pa_{CO_2} with no change in Pa_{CO_2}.

d may be compensated for by increasing F_{IO_2}.

e may be compensated for by increased minute ventilation.

55 **Carbon dioxide retention may cause**
a increase in plasma catecholamine concentrations.
b sweating.
c cardiac arrhythmias.

d constricted pupils.

e decreased cardiac output.

56 **During pregnancy**
a tidal volume increases.
b closing volume increases.
c Pa_{CO_2} is increased in the third trimester.
d progesterone stimulates the respiratory centre.
e the FVC is reduced.

57 **The anterior pituitary gland secretes**
a oxytocin.

b aldosterone.

c thyrotrophin (TSH).

d prolactin (PRL).

e somatostatin (GHRIH).

a **False** Increased $\dot{V}/\dot{Q}$ ratio constitutes increased dead space.
b **True** Shunting would be represented by a decreased $\dot{V}/\dot{Q}$ ratio.
c **False** If minute ventilation remains unchanged, Pa_{CO_2} increases Pa_{O_2} decreases. If alveolar ventilation is maintained by an increase in total minute ventilation, Pa_{CO_2} remains constant but Pa_{O_2} does not decrease.
d **False** Compensation occurs only by an increase in minute ventilation, although the decreased Pa_{O_2} can be overcome by increasing Fi_{O_2}.
e **True** Increased minute ventilation is necessary to maintain alveolar ventilation in the presence of increased physiological dead space.

a **True** Carbon dioxide causes an increase in sympatho-adrenal output.
b **True** Excessive sympatho-adrenal activity causes sweating.
c **True** This results from the release of adrenaline and respiratory acidosis, which accompany carbon dioxide retention.
d **False** Dilated pupils would be expected in the presence of catecholamine secretion.
e **False** Carbon dioxide retention causes an increased cardiac output.

a **True**
b **False** Closing volume does not exceed FRC in normal pregnancy.
c **False** There is a decrease in Pa_{CO_2}.
d **True** This stimulates a 50% increase in minute volume.
e **False** Vital capacity is unchanged.

a **False** Oxytocin is secreted by the posterior pituitary gland (neurohypophysis).
b **False** Aldosterone is an adrenocortical hormone secreted under the influence of the renin–angiotensin system.
c **True** TSH is secreted by the anterior pituitary under the influence of thyrotrophin releasing hormone (TRH).
d **True** PRL is secreted under the inhibitory control of dopamine from the hypothalamus.
e **False** GHRIH is the inhibitory hormone from the hypothalamus which controls growth hormone secretion from the anterior pituitary.

58 The sympathetic nervous system

a does not possess cholinergic fibres.

b releases hormones which may be blocked by guanethidine.

c inhibits motility in the gastrointestinal system.

d produces miosis.

e possesses fibres which run in the vagus nerve.

59 The knee jerk reflex

a is mediated via T12.

b is mediated via afferent impulses from receptors in the patellar tendon.

c is mediated via afferent impulses from receptors in the quadriceps muscle.

d is a monosynaptic reflex.

e disappears under deep general anaesthesia.

60 Myocardial contractility is affected by

a heart rate.

b circulating volume.

c resting length of His–Purkinje fibres.

d parasympathetic activity.

e calcium.

(Ch. 12, A & S)

a **False** Preganglionic sympathetic fibres are cholinergic, as are sympathetic fibres to the sweat glands and some vessels in muscle.

b **True** Guanethidine inhibits release of noradrenaline from postganglionic fibres and also depletes the nerve endings of noradrenaline. It is used in an IVRA technique to produce peripheral sympathetic block.

c **True** Sympathetic stimulation decreases gastrointestinal motility and causes sphincter contraction.

d **False** Sympathetic activity results in pupillary dilation.

e **True** Sympathetic fibres to the heart, bronchi and gut accompany the parasympathetic vagal supply to these organs *(Ch. 4, A & S)*.

(Ch. 14, D)

a **False** The knee jerk reflex is mediated via L3–4.

b **False** Stretching the patellar tendon activates stretch receptors in the quadriceps muscle.

c **True** See **b** above.

d **True** Impulses from the afferent neurons pass directly to the lower motor neurons of the quadriceps muscle.

e **True** Anaesthesia depresses all reflex activity.

(Ch. 2, A & S)

a **False** Heart rate and contractility are usually independent.

b **True** The preload is determined partly by the circulating blood volume. An increased venous return to the heart increases end-diastolic fibre length, and thus myocardial contractility is increased (Frank–Starling relationship).

c **False** The His–Purkinje system is the 'electrical conducting' system of the heart, which transmits the wave of depolarization from the atrioventricular (AV) node into the ventricles.

d **True** Vagal stimulation decreases contractility and also heart rate.

e **True** Calcium ions increase contractility.

61 **A bellows spirometer (e.g. Vitalograph) may be used to measure**

 a   expiratory reserve volume.

 b   closing volume.

 c   total lung capacity.

 d   functional residual capacity.

 e   residual volume.

---

62 **Cerebral blood flow**

 a   is reduced by hyperventilation.
 b   increases if arterial P_{O_2} is less than 7 kPa.
 c   remains stable over a mean arterial pressure range of 60–130 mmHg.

 d   increases with increased JVP.

 e   is dependent on intracranial pressure.

---

63 **Ventilatory minute volume is increased by**

 a   ascent to altitude.

 b   a Pa_{O_2} of 10 kPa.

 c   chronic anaemia.

 d   an $F_{I_{O_2}}$ of 0.03.

 e   inspired CO_2 concentration of 0.03%.

---

64 **In the elderly**

 a FEV_1 is reduced.
 b   cardiac stroke volume is reduced.
 c   physiological dead space is reduced.
 d   GFR is reduced.
 e   FRC exceeds closing volume.

(Appendix VIII, A & S)
a **True** The expiratory reserve volume is that volume which can be exhaled after a normal tidal volume.
b **False** Closing volume is measured usually by the nitrogen washout technique.
c **False** Total lung capacity includes residual volume, and this cannot be measured using simple spirometry.
d **False** Functional residual capacity comprises expiratory reserve volume and residual volume. This is usually determined by means of a dilution technique, using an indicator such as helium.
e **False** Residual volume cannot be measured by simple spirometry (see above).

(Ch. 37, A & S)
a **True** Hypocapnia results in a reduction in cerebral blood flow.
b **True** Hypoxaemia causes a dramatic increase in cerebral blood flow.
c **True** This is the usual autoregulatory range in a normotensive patient.
d **False** Increased jugular venous pressure may reduce cerebral perfusion pressure, and thus cerebral blood flow.
e **True**

(Ch. 1, A & S)
a **True** A reduction in P_{IO_2} leads to a reduction in Pa_{O_2}, with stimulation of peripheral chemoreceptors.
b **False** A Pa_{O_2} of 10 kPa represents the lower limit of the normal range for a healthy individual.
c **False** With chronic anaemia, there is no increase in ventilatory minute volume. However, 2,3-DPG concentration increases and this enhances oxygen-carrying capacity.
d **True** An F_{IO_2} of 0.03 increases ventilatory minute volume transiently, prior to death from hypoxaemia.
e **False** This is the normal concentration of carbon dioxide in the atmosphere.

(Ch. 17, D)
a **True** There is loss of elastic tissue.
b **True** Maximum work rate is therefore restricted.
c **False** Reduced lung elasticity results in increased V_D/V_T.
d **True** This decreases by 1% per annum after 40 years of age.
e **False** Airway closure occurs at the end of a tidal breath, even when erect.

65 During infancy

a ECF volume is proportionately increased compared with adults.
b The larynx is narrowest at the level of the thyroid cartilage.
c The blood volume is approximately 80 ml/kg.
d Oxygen consumption rate is twice that of an adult.
e Ventilation uses up to 15% of oxygen consumption.

66 Bilirubin

a contains products of cytochrome metabolism.

b when unconjugated, is bound to globulin in the plasma.
c is excreted in the bile, mostly as the monoglucuronide.
d appears in excess concentration in the blood in its conjugated form in hepatic disease.
e is not detectable in the urine of healthy patients in its conjugated form.

67 The liver is the major metabolic site of the following:

a insulin.
b glucagon.
c oestrogens.
d thyroxine.
e lignocaine.

68 Cardiac output in a normal subject

a increases with increased CVP.
b increases with increases in metabolic rate.
c increases in pyrexia.
d increases with increase in systemic arterial pressure.

e decreases with raised pulmonary capillary wedge pressure (PCWP).

69 Impulse propagation in a nerve

a is faster in unmyelinated nerves.

b occurs as a result of ionic transfer across the membrane.
c occurs as a result of electrical activity across the membrane.
d may occur at 120 m/s.
e may be slowed by prilocaine.

(Ch. 33, A & S)

a	**True**	ECF/ICF ratio may approach unity in the neonate.
b	**False**	The cricoid cartilage limits the laryngeal diameter.
c	**True**	
d	**True**	It is approximately 6 ml/kg.
e	**True**	This is considerably greater than in the adult (1–2%).

(Ch. 10, D)

a	**True**	20% of bilirubin comprises products of catabolism of enzymes such as cytochromes and peroxidases.
b	**False**	Unconjugated bilirubin is bound to albumin.
c	**False**	80% of bilirubin in bile is the diglucuronide.
d	**True**	Serum bilirubin follows the progress of hepatic disease and its treatment.
e	**True**	

(Ch. 10, D)

a	**True**	
b	**True**	
c	**True**	
d	**False**	Thyroxine undergoes widespread tissue metabolism.
e	**True**	The liver is the main site of drug metabolism.

(Ch. 2, A & S)

a	**True**	This is induced by the Frank–Starling mechanism.
b	**True**	This is a normal physiological response.
c	**True**	
d	**False**	Cardiac output and peripheral resistance together determine systemic arterial pressure.
e	**False**	Cardiac output increases with increased PCWP.

(Ch. 4, A & S)

a	**False**	Myelinated nerves conduct faster than unmyelinated fibres (120 m/s: 0.5–2 m/s).
b	**True**	This is the process of depolarization.
c	**False**	Electrical charges reflect ionic shifts, but do not cause them.
d	**True**	See **a** above.
e	**True**	Local anaesthetic agents block the Na^+/K^+ conduction channels *(Ch. 14, A & S)*.

70 Oxygen

a may cause convulsions at hyperbaric pressure.

b forms an inflammable mixture with air.

c is manufactured by fractional distillation of air.
d has a critical temperature of 36.4°C.

e causes bone marrow depression with prolonged administration.

71 Hyperventilation occurs in response to

a metabolic acidosis.
b high altitude.

c low CSF pH.
d increase in base excess.

e deep sleep.

72 The liver

a receives its blood supply predominantly from the hepatic artery.
b has a blood supply controlled by an autoregulatory mechanism.

c is palpable normally below the right costal margin.

d contains large stores of vitamin K.

e undergoes shrinkage with advancing age and cirrhosis.

73 In a well-oxygenated, otherwise healthy middle-aged man, a Pa_{CO_2}, of 6.1 kPa causes

a pulmonary vasoconstriction.

b cerebral vasodilatation.
c release of catecholamines.

d raised systemic arterial pressure.

e low urinary pH.

(Ch. 8, A & S)

a **True** Convulsions may occur with 100% O_2 at a pressure exceeding 2 atm.

b **False** Although oxygen supports combustion, it is not itself flammable.

c **True** The other major product of this process is nitrogen.

d **False** The critical temperature of oxygen is –118°C; that of nitrous oxide is 36.4°C (Ch. 15, A & S).

e **False** Nitrous oxide causes bone marrow depression after prolonged use.

(Ch. 1, A & S)

a **True**

b **True** At high altitude, the reduction in F_{IO_2} leads to hypoxaemia; unacclimatized subjects respond to this by hyperventilation.

c **True** This stimulates the central chemoreceptors.

d **False** An increase in base excess accompanies alkalosis or decreased hydrogen ion concentration.

e **False** The normal response to deep sleep is hypoventilation. Sleep apnoea syndrome represents a severe form of this.

(Ch. 10, D)

a **False** The portal vein supplies approximately 60% of liver blood flow.

b **True** Hepatic arterial flow may compensate for variations in portal venous flow.

c **True** Normally, there is descent of the liver on inspiration and the liver is palpable on deep inspiration.

d **False** Storage capacity for vitamin K is small, in contrast to that for vitamins D and B_{12}.

e **True** Liver reserve is reduced in the elderly and in later stages of cirrhosis.

(Ch. 4, D)

a **False** Pulmonary vasoconstriction is usually mediated via hypoxaemia.

b **True**

c **True** The sweaty, flushed appearance of hypercapnic patients is caused by release of catecholamines.

d **True** Catecholamine release causes an increase in systemic arterial pressure.

e **True** The kidneys compensate for respiratory acidosis by excreting acid (Ch. 21, A & S).

74 **The following are true of albumin:**
   a   It has a molecular weight of 70 000 daltons.

   b   Its plasma concentration is usually 35–50 g/l.

   c   Hyperalbuminaemia occurs in liver failure.
   d   It has an important transport role.

   e   It is excreted in excess in nephrotic syndrome.

---

75 **In the peripheral blood**
   a   normally, about 3% of total oxygen content is carried as dissolved oxygen.
   b Pa_{O_2} is normally the same as PA_{O_2}.

   c   arterial P_{CO_2} is determined solely by the minute ventilation.

   d   carbon dioxide is transported largely as bicarbonate.

   e   whilst breathing air, the partial pressure of nitrogen is the same in arterial as in venous blood.

---

76 **With respect to the control of ventilation**
   a   the chemoreceptors in the carotid and aortic bodies are stimulated by anaemia.
   b   marked respiratory stimulation occurs when F_{IO_2} < 60 mmHg.

   c   hypoxaemia increases the ventilatory response to hypercapnia.

   d   when Pa_{CO_2} chronically exceeds Pa_{O_2}, the respiratory centre is depressed by hypercapnia.
   e   afferents from the carotid bodies ascend to the medulla via the vagus nerve.

---

77 **Effects of hypercapnia include**
   a   coma when Pa_{CO_2} exceeds 10 kPa.
   b   a reduction in sympathetic tone.

   c   an increase in serum potassium concentration.

   d   an increase in CSF pressure.
   e   potentiation of depolarizing relaxants.

a	**True**	The average molecular weight of albumin is approximately 70 000 daltons.
b	**True**	This is the normal plasma concentration of albumin *(Appendix IV, A & S)*.
c	**False**	Liver failure is characterized by hypoalbuminaemia *(Ch. 10, D)*.
d	**True**	Many drugs undergo protein binding, which facilitates rapid distribution in vivo *(Ch. 7, A & S)*.
e	**True**	Hypoproteinaemic oedema occurs in nephrotic syndrome, secondary to albumin loss *(Ch. 6, D)*.

(Ch. 1, A & S)

a	**False**	Approximately 1.5% of the oxygen content of arterial blood is dissolved in plasma, normally.
b	**False**	There is normally a small alveolar–arterial partial pressure difference, because of the presence of physiological shunting and $\dot{V}/\dot{Q}$ scatter.
c	**False**	Arterial P_{CO_2} is determined by CO_2 production and minute ventilation.
d	**True**	Carbonic acid dissociation in the red blood cell liberates bicarbonate ions, which diffuse into the plasma.
e	**True**	Tissues do not produce nitrogen.

(Ch. 1, A & S)

a	**False**	Peripheral chemoreceptors respond to Pa_{O_2}, and not oxygen content or haemoglobin concentration.
b	**False**	Respiratory stimulation occurs when Pa_{O_2} is less than 60 mmHg (8 kPa). $F_{I_{O_2}}$ is the inspired fractional concentration of oxygen.
c	**True**	The slope of the carbon dioxide response curve is increased in the presence of hypoxaemia.
d	**True**	Care should be exercised during administration of postoperative oxygen therapy.
e	**False**	The carotid sinus nerve is a branch of the glossopharyngeal nerve.

(Ch. 4, D)

a	**True**	Drowsiness and coma supervene with severe hypercapnia.
b	**False**	Hypercapnia stimulates the sympathetic nervous system and cardiac output is increased.
c	**True**	Hypercapnia leads to acidosis and favours movement of intracellular potassium into the extracellular fluid *(Ch. 21, A & S)*.
d	**True**	Carbon dioxide is a potent vasodilator.
e	**False**	There is no potentiation of neuromuscular block.

78 Central venous pressure
a always represents left atrial pressure.

b decreases with the onset of tachycardia in the healthy young patient.
c increases with fluid overload.
d may be 5 mmHg in the normal individual.
e may be measured in the inferior vena cava.

79 The following are neurotransmitters at autonomic ganglia:
a adrenaline.
b noradrenaline.

c dopamine.

d 5-HT.

e acetylcholine.

80 The following changes tend to occur postoperatively:
a hypoglycaemia.

b decreased K^+ excretion.

c increased production of cortisol.

d increased production of adrenaline.

e raised serum concentration of ADH.

81 In respect of the ABO blood groups
a these are inherited in Mendelian fashion.
b a patient with group AB has anti-A and anti-B antibodies.

c antibodies are found in saliva.
d blood may be typed independently if anti-A and anti-B sera are available.
e group AB is the universal recipient.

(Chs. 2 and 20, A & S)

a **False** Central venous pressure reflects right atrial pressure. It reflects left atrial pressure only in the absence of pulmonary hypertension, mitral valve disease, etc. In these situations, pulmonary capillary wedge pressure is a better indicator of left atrial pressure.
b **True** There is a transient decrease in central venous pressure with the onset of tachycardia.
c **True** This is an early sign of fluid overload.
d **True** The normal range for central venous pressure is 0–8 mmHg.
e **True** Provided that the end of the measuring catheter is intrathoracic.

(Ch. 4, A & S)

a **False**
b **False** Noradrenaline is the postganglionic neurotransmitter in most of the sympathetic nervous system.
c **False** Dopamine is a neurotransmitter at central sites, but not at peripheral ganglia.
d **False** 5-HT is a central neurotransmitter found in the brain stem and spinal cord.
e **True**

(Ch. 21, A & S)

a **False** The sympatho-adrenal response to surgery and stress involves mobilization of glucose via gluconeogenesis and glycogenolysis.
b **False** Increased secretion of cortisol and aldosterone results in sodium and water retention and potassium excretion.
c **True** This is part of the endocrine response to stress and surgery. Steroid-treated patients must receive perioperative replacement therapy.
d **True** Increased sympatho-adrenal activity is part of the stress response to surgery.
e **True** ADH is secreted in response to stress, augmenting the water retention which occurs postoperatively.

(Ch. 6, A & S)

a **True** In the UK, 47% of persons are group O.
b **False** Group AB has neither anti-A nor anti-B antibodies in the serum.
c **True** Antibodies in saliva give an indication of the ABO blood group.
d **True** This is the basis of blood grouping tests.
e **True** Group AB has no serum antibodies.

82 **Increased vagal activity results in**
a reduced rate of depolarization of the cardiac muscle.
b reduced sinoatrial (SA) nodal activity.
c reduced atrioventricular (AV) nodal activity.
d raised threshold potential.
e changes in potassium permeability.

83 **The following factors increase production of renin:**
a reduction in renal perfusion pressure.

b increased intracellular $[Na^+]$ and decreased extracellular $[K^+]$.

c angiotensin II.

d decreased plasma volume.

e lumbar extradural block.

84 **The following values for water distribution are correct for a 70 kg man:**
a total body water (TBW) = 49 l.

b intracellular fuid (ICF) = 28 l.
c extracellular fluid (ECF) = 21 l.
d plasma volume = 3.5 l.
e interstitial fluid = 3.5 l.

85 **ADH production**
a is stimulated by morphine and ether.

b is under hypothalamic control.
c is stimulated by increase in plasma osmolality.

d is inhibited by decrease in plasma volume.

e is inhibited by ethanol.

(Ch. 2, A & S)

a	**True**	
b	**True**	
c	**False**	There is no vagal innervation of the AV node.
d	**False**	The threshold potential of –50 mV is unaffected.
e	**False**	Changes in potassium permeability affect the resting membrane potential. This is unaffected by vagal activity.

(Ch. 3, A & S)

a	**True**	A baroreceptor mechanism in the afferent arteriole detects a decrease in renal blood flow.
b	**False**	Increased secretion of renin and aldosterone is caused by a decrease in extracellular sodium concentration or increased extracellular potassium concentration.
c	**False**	Angiotensin II is part of the pathway between renin and the stimulation of aldosterone secretion. Angiotensin II suppresses secretion of renin.
d	**True**	A reduction in plasma volume results in reduction in renal perfusion pressure.
e	**True**	Sympathetic block results in hypotension and decreased renal perfusion pressure.

(Appendix VI and Ch. 3, A & S)

a	**False**	Total body water is 60% of body weight, which would be 42 l in a 70 kg man.
b	**True**	Intracellular fluid volume is two-thirds of the total body water.
c	**False**	Extracellular fluid volume would amount to 14 l.
d	**True**	Plasma volume is 50 ml/kg in an adult.
e	**False**	Interstitial fluid volume is ECF minus plasma volume, i.e. approximately 10.5 l.

(Ch. 8, D)

a	**True**	ADH release may be stimulated by drugs such as morphine, phenothiazines and tricyclic antidepressants. Ether has sympathomimetic actions and may stimulate ADH release.
b	**True**	Osmoreceptors are situated in the hypothalamus *(Ch. 3, A & S)*.
c	**True**	An increase in plasma osmolality stimulates the synthesis of ADH in the supraoptic nuclei.
d	**False**	A 15% decrease in plasma volume with no change in osmolality stimulates secretion of ADH.
e	**True**	This accounts for the diuretic effect of alcohol.

86 The following are associated with sodium retention:

a congestive cardiac failure.

b hepatic failure.

c infusion of hypotonic fluid.

d excessive sweating.

e oedema.

87 Pulmonary function tests in a 25-year-old female of 58 kg reveal FEV_1 2.45 l, FVC 3.0 l. These may indicate

a a diagnosis of asthma.

b the patient is asymptomatic.

c the need for an urgent ventilation/perfusion scan.
d myasthenia gravis.

e hyperventilation.

88 Ingestion of 20 ml/kg water over a period of 20 min normally results in

a increased urine output for 12 h.

b reduction in interstitial fluid osmolality.

c increased secretion of ADH.

d stimulation of carotid sinus receptors.

e increase in atrial natriuretic hormone production.

a **True** Stimulation of intra-arterial receptors results in sodium retention *(Ch. 5, D)*.

b **True** In hepatic failure, hormone metabolism is impaired and the actions of aldosterone are prolonged *(Ch. 5, D)*.

c **False** After infusion of a hypotonic fluid, some sodium is excreted with the excess water.

d **False** Excess sweat contains little sodium and does not alter sodium homeostasis significantly.

e **True** Oedema is frequently associated with sodium retention *(Ch. 3, D)*.

(Appendix VIII, A & S)

a **False** The FEV_1/FVC ratio is normal (approximately 80%). In asthma, this ratio is reduced.

b **True** These values are normal for a 25-year-old female of short stature.

c **False** See **b** above.

d **True** These values may be found in a well-controlled myasthenic. However, both FEV_1 and FVC may be reduced greatly in an undiagnosed or poorly-controlled myasthenic patient *(Ch. 40, A & S)*.

e **False** Pulmonary function tests do not give any indication of rate of ventilation or tidal volume.

(Ch. 21, A & S; Ch. 5, D)

a **False** The increased urine output resulting from ingestion of 1.4 l by a 70 kg man would last for approximately 1–2 h.

b **True** This water load would lead to a reduction in interstitial fluid osmolality.

c **False** ADH secretion would be increased in the presence of dehydration or increased interstitial fluid osmolality.

d **False** The carotid sinus receptors respond to increased arterial pressure. Changes in plasma volume are sensed by atrial (predominantly right) volume receptors.

e **True** Stimulation of the atrial stretch receptors increases production of atrial natriuretic hormone *(Ch. 3, A & S)*.

89 In the full term neonate

a pulmonary arterial pressure declines in the first 2 weeks.

b the oxyhaemoglobin dissociation curve is shifted to the right.

c unconjugated jaundice is common during the first week.

d approximately 80% of haemoglobin is HbF.

e vitamin K should be administered to counteract the development of jaundice.

90 In the renal tubule

a almost 95% of the glomerular filtrate is reabsorbed.

b 65% of sodium is absorbed in the proximal convoluted tubule (PCT).

c aldosterone increases sodium absorption in the PCT.

d hydrogen ions are excreted mostly as phosphate.

e arginine vasopressin increases water permeability in the collecting ducts.

91 Cardiac output

a is the product of heart rate and systemic vascular resistance.

b may be measured by the Fick principle.

c may be measured by a technique involving 5% glucose.

d increase is always accompanied by increased oxygen consumption.

e is reduced more by isoflurane than by halothane.

92 The first rib

a is grooved by the subclavian vein.

b articulates with the body of the sternum.

c is the insertion for scalenus anterior.

d is crossed by the cords of the brachial plexus.

e forms part of the thoracic inlet.

a **True** There is a rapid decline from fetal values at first, then a gradual reduction to reach adult values after 2 weeks.
b **False** The presence of HbF shifts the curve to the left.
c **True** This is more likely in the presence of hypoglycaemia and hypothermia, and is treated by phototherapy.
d **True** The subsequent decline in production of HbF, with conversion to synthesis of HbA, contributes to the physiological anaemia of infancy.
e **False** Vitamin K is given to supplement the neonatal hepatic stores and to promote synthesis of coagulation factors.

a **False** Approximately 99% of glomerular filtrate is reabsorbed.
b **True** Active transport in combination with passive transport accounts for absorption of the majority of filtered sodium at this site.
c **False** Aldosterone increases sodium absorption in the distal convoluted tubule and the collecting duct.
d **False** Hydrogen ions are excreted in combination with ammonia (67%) and phosphate (33%).
e **True** Arginine vasopressin is ADH and is secreted in response to increased extracellular fluid osmolality.

a **False** Cardiac output is the product of heart rate and stroke volume.
b **True** This is the standard method of measurement; cardiac output is equal to oxygen consumption divided by the arteriovenous oxygen content difference.
c **True** In the thermodilution technique, cold glucose is injected into the right atrium and temperature change measured in the pulmonary artery.
d **False** Increases in cardiac output may occur without an increase in oxygen consumption.
e **False** Halothane reduces myocardial contractility to a greater extent than does isoflurane *(Ch. 8, A & S)*.

a **True** The vein runs anterior to the artery and brachial plexus.
b **False** The first rib articulates with the manubrium sterni.
c **True** The scalenus anterior muscle is inserted between the subclavian artery and vein.
d **False** The cords of the brachial plexus surround the axillary artery. The roots of the brachial plexus lie behind the scalenus anterior and the trunks emerge from its lateral border.
e **True** Together with T1 and the manubrium sterni.

93   In the normal heart
   a   the right ventricle contracts before the left.

   b   the right atrium contracts before the left atrium.
   c   the interventricular septum depolarizes from left to right.

   d   the normal PR interval is 0.22 s.

   e   the refractory period of cardiac muscle is 0.5 s.

94   Coagulation of blood
   a   initially involves the aggregation of platelets at the point of
       vessel damage.
   b   involves the production of thrombin from factor II.

   c   occurs under the influence of either an intrinsic system or an
       extrinsic cascade.
   d   is impaired in haemophilia B as a result of deficiency of factor
       IX.
   e   is inhibited by activation of antithrombin III by heparin.

95   Intraocular pressure (IOP) is
   a   less than atmospheric pressure when the globe is open.

   b   decreased by halothane.

   c   decreased by a 15° head-up tilt.

   d   increased throughout the duration of a Valsalva manoeuvre.

   e   increased by hypercapnia.

**96   Dilatation of the blood vessels in the skin of the left hand may be
       caused by**
   a   halothane.

   b   nitric oxide
   c   immersing the right hand in hot water.

   d   drinking 500 ml of warm milk.
   e   hyperventilation.

(Ch. 2, A & S)

a **False** The right atrium contracts before the left atrium but the ventricles normally contract synchronously.
b **True** See **a** above.
c **True** The bundle of His supplying the left ventricle depolarizes first. This leads to the initial Q wave of a ventricular depolarization.
d **False** The normal PR interval is 0.12–0.2 s. An interval of 0.22 s indicates first degree heart block *(Appendix IIIa, A & S)*.
e **False** The refractory period is normally less than 0.3 s.

(Ch. 6, A & S; Ch. 11, D)

a **False** The initial action is vessel spasm and platelet adhesion.

b **True** Prothrombin (factor II) is converted to thrombin under the influence of activated factor X.
c **True** The intrinsic system is more potent. Both systems result in activation of factor X.
d **True** Factor IX (Christmas factor) deficiency leads to a similar clinical picture to classical haemophilia.
e **False** Antithrombin III is a naturally occurring thrombin inactivator, which is potentiated by heparin.

(Ch. 28, A & S)

a **False** When the globe is opened, intraocular pressure becomes the same as atmospheric pressure.
b **True** Halothane, in common with other volatile anaesthetic agents, decreases intraocular pressure.
c **True** Intraocular pressure is dependent upon central venous pressure, which is reduced by a 15° head-up tilt.
d **False** Although there is a transient increase in intraocular pressure with increased intrathoracic pressure, the adaptive mechanism counteracts any sustained rise.
e **True** There is a linear relationship between intraocular pressure and arterial carbon dioxide tension.

(Ch. 2, A & S)

a **True** Peripheral vasodilatation is a feature of spontaneous ventilation with halothane. If Pa_{CO_2} is controlled, halothane has no effect.
b **True** This occurs via cyclic AMP.
c **True** There is a direct and consensual component to vasodilatation with hot water immersion.
d **True** Although the effect may be transient!
e **False** Hyperventilation is associated with peripheral vasoconstriction as a result of hypocapnia.

97 **In the normal lungs**

    a inspiration of 100% O_2 may dilate pulmonary blood vessels.

    b ventilation is greater at the apex of the lung.

    c 5-HT causes an increase in bronchial resistance.
    d histamine increases the pulmonary arterial pressure.

    e noradrenaline increases pulmonary vascular resistance.

98 **The following are used in indicator dilution methods to measure cardiac output:**

    a indocyanine green.

    b Fick principle.

    c Cuvette densitometer.

    d interferometer.

    e polarography.

99 **The following may prolong gastric emptying:**

    a atropine.
    b metoclopramide.
    c morphine.

    d cimetidine.

    e nalbuphine.

100 **In respect of the cardiovascular system during pregnancy**

    a cardiac output increases in the first trimester.

    b peripheral resistance is unaltered.

    c venous return is obstructed in the supine position after the 13th week.
    d pulmonary vascularity appears increased on chest X-radiographs.

    e circulation time is decreased.

(Ch. 1, A & S)

a **True** Hypoxic pulmonary vasoconstriction is abolished by inspiration of 100% oxygen *(Ch. 38, A & S)*.

b **False** Ventilation per unit volume is 50% greater at the base of the lung.

c **True** 5-HT causes bronchoconstriction *(Ch. 22, A & S)*.

d **True** Histamine produces pulmonary vasoconstriction but peripheral vasodilatation.

e **True** Noradrenaline causes pulmonary vasoconstriction.

(Ch. 2, A & S)

a **True** Indocyanine green is the indicator used normally in dye dilution methods.

b **False** This may be used to measure cardiac output but is not the principle underlying indicator dilution methods.

c **True** The Cuvette densitometer is used in the measurement of indocyanine green concentration; sampling is usually from the radial artery.

d **False** An interferometer is used to measure gas concentration, e.g. in the calibration of vaporizers.

e **False** Polarography is a method of measuring oxygen concentration.

(Ch. 7, A & S)

a **True**

b **False** Metoclopramide increases gastric motility *(Ch. 13, A & S)*.

c **True** Morphine reduces gastrointestinal motility, and delays gastric emptying in particular.

d **False** Cimetidine has no effect on gastric emptying or gastrointestinal motility.

e **True** Nalbuphine is an opioid analgesic and delays gastric emptying.

(Ch. 5, A & S)

a **True** Contractility, heart rate and stroke volume increase, resulting in an increase of approximately 1.5 l/min.

b **False** Peripheral resistance decreases in mid-trimester because of new vessel formation and reduced vascular tone.

c **True** The supine hypotensive syndrome may occur after the beginning of the second trimester.

d **True** Pulmonary blood flow is increased, and this is evident as increased vascularity in the chest X-radiograph.

e **False** There is no significant change in circulation time.

2. Pharmacology

1   **A highly ionized drug**
   a   is well absorbed from the intestine.

   b   is excreted mainly in the kidney.

   c   crosses the placenta easily.
   d   is reabsorbed from the renal tubule.

   e   is highly protein-bound.

2   **Sodium nitroprusside decreases arterial pressure by**
   a   an action on alpha-receptors.

   b   reducing cardiac output.

   c   causing bradycardia.

   d   producing cyanide ions.

   e   a direct action on blood vessels.

3   **The following are eliminated by the kidney mainly in the unchanged form:**
   a   vecuronium.

   b   suxamethonium.

   c   dopamine.
   d   doxacurium.
   e   digoxin.

(Ch. 7, A & S)

a **False** The undissociated moiety of a drug crosses membranes in the gastrointestinal tract. Highly ionized drugs are less well absorbed.
b **True** Highly ionized drugs are water soluble and are excreted readily by the kidney.
c **False** Drugs in the ionized form are poorly lipid-soluble.
d **False** The p*K*a and acidity of the filtrate determine the extent of ionization within the renal tubules, but in general terms, ionized drugs are reabsorbed poorly at this site.
e **False** Highly lipid-soluble drugs undergo protein binding to a greater extent than ionized drugs, which are freely soluble in plasma.

(Ch. 36, A & S)

a **False** Sodium nitroprusside is a direct-acting vasodilator, and does not act via adrenoceptors.
b **False** Nitroprusside affects predominantly resistance vessels, and has no direct effect on cardiac contractility.
c **False** Hypotension induced by nitroprusside is accompanied by reflex tachycardia.
d **False** Nitroprusside is metabolized to cyanide ions, which may reach toxic concentrations after prolonged administration. However, this is not related to its hypotensive action.
e **True**

(Ch. 11, A & S)

a **False** Vecuronium is metabolized by the liver and excreted in the bile.
b **False** Suxamethonium undergoes ester hydrolysis by plasma cholinesterases.
c **False** Dopamine is metabolized extensively throughout the body.
d **True** A small amount (6%) of metabolism by cholinesterase occurs.
e **True** Digoxin should be administered with reduced frequency in the presence of renal impairment *(Ch. 13, A & S)*.

4 **Edrophonium is used for**
  a testing for the presence of myasthenia gravis.
  b antagonism of neuromuscular blockade.

  c producing central respiratory stimulation.

  d relief of urinary retention.

  e treatment of myotonia congenita.

5 **Morphine administered extradurally**
  a may cause intense itching.
  b may cause urinary retention.
  c may produce nausea and vomiting.

  d leads to delayed respiratory depression not relieved by naloxone.
  e acts by binding to receptors in the postcentral gyrus.

6 **An untoward reaction to the following may occur in a patient taking monoamine oxidase inhibitors (MAOIs):**
  a adrenaline.

  b thiopentone.
  c diazepam.
  d tricyclic antidepressants.

  e amphetamine.

7 **Nitrous oxide**
  a increases cardiac output.
  b decreases peripheral resistance.

  c causes no significant change in arterial blood pressure in healthy individuals.
  d increases heart rate.
  e sensitizes the heart to exogenous catecholamines.

(Ch. 11, A & S)

a	**True**	This is described as the Tensilon test *(Ch. 14, D)*.
b	**True**	Edrophonium is an anticholinesterase, and may be used for this purpose.
c	**False**	Edrophonium does not possess respiratory stimulant properties.
d	**False**	An anticholinesterase may be effective in relieving urinary retention. However, edrophonium is not used commonly for this purpose.
e	**False**	It is not used for the treatment of this condition.

(Ch. 10, A & S)

a	**True**	This is a commonly reported side-effect.
b	**True**	Urinary retention is a common side-effect.
c	**True**	Nausea and vomiting occur as frequently as with other routes of administration.
d	**False**	Naloxone antagonizes respiratory depression associated with extradural morphine.
e	**False**	Spinal opioid receptors are located in the substantia gelatinosa.

(Ch. 29, A & S)

a	**True**	Augmentation of the action of adrenaline and other sympathomimetics occurs in the presence of MAOI drugs.
b	**False**	Thiopentone has no sympathomimetic activity.
c	**False**	Diazepam has no sympathomimetic activity.
d	**False**	However, the combination of tricyclic and MAOI antidepressants should be used with extreme caution.
e	**True**	Amphetamine is a sympathomimetic agent; hypertensive crisis may occur with the combination *(Appendix 1, BNF)*.

(Ch. 8, A & S)

a	**False**	Cardiac output is depressed.
b	**False**	Peripheral resistance is increased; in combination with **a** above, there is little change in arterial pressure in healthy individuals.
c	**True**	See **b** above.
d	**False**	There is little effect on heart rate.
e	**False**	This is true of halothane, but not nitrous oxide.

8 Halothane

a increases GI tract motility.
b increases cerebral blood flow.
c is metabolized to an extent of 10% of the administered dose.
d increases cerebral metabolic rate.
e increases intraocular pressure.

9 Enflurane

a is an ether.
b is inflammable but not explosive in concentrations greater than 4% in oxygen.
c has the formula: $CHBrClCF_3$.
d is metabolized to yield free bromide ions.
e is metabolized to yield free fluoride ions.

10 Ketamine

a has antanalgesic properties.
b is an antisialogogue.

c increases heart rate.
d must be given intramuscularly.
e may cause unpleasant dreams in children.

11 Depolarizing neuromuscular block is associated with

a fasciculations.
b fade on tetanic stimulation.
c enhancement by volatile agents.
d antagonism by anticholinesterase drugs.
e postoperative myalgia.

12 Factors which determine the rate of increase of alveolar concentration of a volatile agent include

a the biotransformation of the agent.
b minute ventilation.

c the MAC of the agent.
d the inspired concentration of the agent.

e cardiac output.

(Chs. 8 and 37, A & S)

a	False	GI motility is depressed, as with other volatile agents.
b	True	Halothane causes cerebral vasodilatation.
c	False	20% of an administered dose undergoes hepatic metabolism.
d	False	Cerebral metabolic rate is decreased.
e	False	Intraocular pressure is decreased.

(Ch. 8, A & S)

a	True	Enflurane is 2-chloro-1,1,2-trifluoroethyl difluoromethyl ether.
b	False	Enflurane is inflammable at concentrations greater than 6% in oxygen.
c	False	This is halothane (see **a** above).
d	False	Enflurane contains no bromine.
e	True	Free fluoride is produced, but not in sufficient concentration to cause renal damage.

(Ch. 9, A & S)

a	False	It has analgesic properties at subanaesthetic concentrations.
b	False	It may cause intense salivation, and premedication with atropine is recommended.
c	True	Heart rate is increased by facilitation of calcium transport.
d	False	It may be given intravenously.
e	True	But children complain less than do adults.

(Ch. 11, A & S)

a	True	This is a characteristic of depolarizing block.
b	False	This is a characteristic of non-depolarizing block.
c	False	This is a characteristic of non-depolarizing block.
d	False	Anticholinesterases may prolong the block.
e	True	This is more prevalent in young ambulant patients.

(Ch. 7, A & S)

a	False	Biotransformation has virtually no influence.
b	True	The rate of increase is determined by the balance between input to, and uptake from, the lungs. For a given inspired concentration, an increase in minute ventilation increases rate of input.
c	False	MAC has no influence; it is a measure of potency.
d	True	Increasing the inspired concentration increases alveolar concentration for a given minute volume.
e	True	The relationship is inverse.

13 Lignocaine

a may be used for treatment of ventricular arrhythmias.

b is used for epidural analgesia in a 4% solution.

c may cause methaemoglobinaemia.
d should be used with special care in patients taking propranolol.

e was first used for i.v. regional analgesia in 1908 by Augustus Bier.

14 Suxamethonium

a acts as an antagonist at the neuromuscular junction.
b is metabolized by hydrolysis.
c hyperpolarizes the transmembrane potential at the neuromuscular junction.
d acts by increasing the flux of sodium and potassium ions.
e antagonizes tubocurarine.

15 Atropine

a completely blocks the vagus nerve in a dose of 0.4 mg/70 kg.
b may cause bradycardia in very low dosage.
c increases physiological dead space.
d produces moderate CNS depression.
e causes pupillary constriction.

16 Isoprenaline

a stimulates the baroreceptors, resulting in bradycardia.
b produces transient bronchospasm.
c is used in a dose of 1–20 µg/min in adults to produce a positive inotropic effect.
d may be used for treatment of complete heart block.
e may cause hypotension because of action at alpha-adrenoceptors.

(Ch. 14, A & S)

a	**True**	It possesses membrane stabilizing properties (Class I anti-arrhythmic) *(Ch. 13, A & S)*.
b	**False**	The maximum recommended dose (200 mg) would be reached with 5 ml of 4% solution.
c	**False**	Prilocaine possesses this side-effect.
d	**True**	Reduction in maintenance therapy of anti-arrhythmics is recommended *(Ch. 13, A & S)*.
e	**False**	Lignocaine was synthesized first in 1948: Bier used procaine.

(Ch. 11, A & S)

a	**False**	Suxamethonium is an agonist, and causes depolarizing block.
b	**True**	Ester hydrolysis by plasma cholinesterase.
c	**False**	The membrane is depolarized, not hyperpolarized.
d	**True**	This is how depolarization occurs.
e	**True**	This represents interaction between a competitive antagonist (dTC, dextrotubocurarine) and a drug which depolarizes the neuromuscular junction, i.e. an agonist.

(Ch. 12, A & S)

a	**False**	A dose greater than this would be required.
b	**True**	This may occur on i.v. administration.
c	**True**	This is caused by vagal blockade and bronchodilation.
d	**False**	Atropine may produce CNS excitation.
e	**False**	Atropine is a mydriatic agent.

(Ch. 12, A & S)

a	**False**	Beta-stimulation causes tachycardia.
b	**False**	Beta-stimulation results in bronchodilation.
c	**True**	0.02–0.40 µg/kg per minute is the recommended dose *(Appendix IIIb, A & S)*.
d	**True**	This is one of the main indications for its use.
e	**False**	Isoprenaline has no alpha-adrenoceptor activity; diastolic arterial pressure may be reduced because of beta-effects on muscle blood vessels (vasodilatation), but systolic pressure is increased by a positive inotropic action.

17 Tricyclic antidepressants
a depress the formation of noradrenaline.
b may cause hypertension.

c may cause arrhythmias.

d may cause renal failure after prolonged administration.
e may produce sedation.

18 Thiopentone
a 2.5% in aqueous solution has a pH of approximately 11.
b is metabolized only by the kidney.
c is an oxybarbiturate.
d is stable in solution for 24 h.

e may be used in a 10% solution.

19 The response to an agonist drug
a occurs as a result of its high affinity (binding) and high intrinsic activity.
b may be antagonized with no change in its receptor affinity.

c may be antagonized competitively by a drug with high intrinsic activity.
d is maximal at low concentrations if it is a partial agonist.

e is a pharmacodynamic property of the drug.

20 The following drugs may be used i.v. in anaesthetic practice for induced hypotension:
a hydralazine.

b captopril.

c sodium nitroprusside.
d glyceryl trinitrate.

e trimetaphan.

(Ch. 29, A & S)

a	**False**	Noradrenaline re-uptake is inhibited.
b	**True**	These drugs should be given with caution to patients with heart disease.
c	**True**	Because of anticholinergic and sympathomimetic effects, overdosage may result in serious and intractable arrhythmias.
d	**False**	This is not a recognized side-effect in therapeutic doses.
e	**True**	

(Ch. 9, A & S)

a	**True**	
b	**False**	Thiopentone undergoes hepatic metabolism.
c	**False**	It is a thiobarbiturate. Pentobarbitone is its oxy-analogue.
d	**True**	And probably longer, but its use after 24 h is not recommended.
e	**True**	But only for rectal administration. Solutions stronger than 2.5% should never be used i.v. because of the risk of tissue damage associated with extravascular leakage.

(Ch. 7, A & S)

a	**True**	An agent with high affinity but no intrinsic activity is an antagonist.
b	**True**	This is non-competitive antagonism. No increase in agonist concentration will overcome the antagonism.
c	**False**	An antagonist binds to receptors but has no intrinsic activity.
d	**False**	A partial agonist is unable to produce a maximal response, even at high concentrations.
e	**True**	

(Ch. 36, A & S)

a	**True**	Hydralazine is a direct acting vasodilator with a slow onset of action.
b	**False**	Captopril is an angiotensin-converting enzyme inhibitor, which has been used as oral pretreatment before hypotensive anaesthesia.
c	**True**	It is a vasodilator which acts directly on blood vessel walls.
d	**True**	Glyceryl trinitrate has direct actions, predominantly on the venous side of the circulation.
e	**True**	Trimetaphan is a sympathetic ganglion blocker, with a short duration of action.

21 The following agents cross the blood–brain barrier:
a tubocurarine.
b hexamethonium.
c lignocaine.

d hyoscine hydrobromide.
e sulphadimidine.

22 The following statements are true:
a Cimetidine potentiates the effects of warfarin.
b Erythromycin potentiates the effects of theophylline.
c Isoflurane potentiates the effects of pancuronium.
d Rifampicin potentiates the effects of glucocorticoids.

e Propranolol antagonizes the effects of verapamil.

23 Dopamine
a crosses the blood–brain barrier.
b is a precursor of L-dopa.

c increases renal blood flow in low dose.

d is ineffective orally.
e causes coronary vasoconstriction.

24 Etomidate
a is excreted unchanged by the kidneys.

b is dissolved in propylene glycol.
c decreases intraocular pressure.
d causes more venous sequelae than thiopentone.

e suppresses adrenocortical function.

(Ch. 7, A & S)

a **False** This is a polar molecule, and poorly lipid-soluble.
b **False** Hexamethonium, a ganglion blocker, is also a polar molecule.
c **True** The undissociated form of lignocaine (free base) is lipid-soluble and free to cross the blood–brain barrier.
d **True** Hyoscine may cause CNS depression, especially in the elderly.
e **True** Sulphonamides are effective in the treatment of meningococcal meningitis (Ch. 14, D).

(Appendix 1, BNF)

a **True**
b **True** This may result in theophylline toxicity.
c **True** (Ch. 8, A & S)
d **False** Rifampicin is an anti-tuberculous drug which causes liver enzyme induction.
e **False** Verapamil is not recommended in combination with a beta-adrenergic blocker.

(Ch. 12, A & S)

a **False**
b **False** Tyrosine is oxidized to L-dopa, and this is decarboxylated to dopamine. Dopamine is a precursor of noradrenaline and adrenaline.
c **True** In a dose of up to 5 µg/kg per minute, the major effect of dopamine is on the renal vasculature.
d **True** Dopamine is given by i.v. infusion.
e **False** But in high doses (greater than 15 µg/kg per minute) peripheral vasoconstriction occurs.

(Ch. 9, A & S)

a **True** Although a small proportion of etomidate is excreted unchanged, the majority is broken down rapidly by hydrolysis.
b **True** It is dissolved in water with 35% propylene glycol at pH 8.1.
c **True** This is true of all i.v. anaesthetic agents except ketamine.
d **True** Pain on injection occurs in up to 80% of patients; this may be minimized by rapid injection into a large vein.
e **True** By suppression of 11-beta-hydroxylase.

25 Which of the following are alpha-blockers?
a phentolamine.

b oxprenolol.
c phenoxybenzamine.

d labetalol.

e prazosin.

26 Digoxin
a causes bronchoconstriction.
b decreases central venous pressure.
c enhances appetite.
d increases pulmonary artery pressure.
e increases urine output.

27 Epileptiform activity may be seen after the following:
a propofol.

b halothane.
c bupivacaine.

d enflurane.

e hypoxaemia.

28 Dantrolene
a is formulated in acidic solution.

b may only be given i.v.

c decreases release of calcium at the sarcoplasmic reticulum.

d causes abnormal liver function tests.

e does not affect the neuromuscular junction.

(Ch. 12, A & S)
a **True** Phentolamine is a short-acting alpha-adrenoceptor blocking drug.
b **False** Oxprenolol is a beta-adrenoceptor blocking drug.
c **True** Phenoxybenzamine is a relatively long-acting alpha-adrenoceptor blocking drug.
d **True** Labetalol is a combined alpha- and beta-blocker, with a relative alpha-blockade:beta-blockade activity of 3:7.
e **True** Prazosin is a postsynaptic alpha-blocking agent with vasodilator properties.

(Ch. 13, A & S)
a **False**
b **True** Secondary to positive inotropic effects.
c **False** Loss of appetite is a common feature.
d **False** Digoxin has no direct effect upon pulmonary vessels.
e **True** Secondary to improved cardiac output.

a **True** There have been reports of seizure activity associated with propofol, although it reduces duration of seizure during ECT *(Ch. 9, A & S)*.
b **False**
c **True** Toxic levels of bupivacaine may cause CNS depression and epileptiform activity *(Ch. 14, A & S)*.
d **True** Enflurane is associated with epileptiform activity on EEG if more than 3% has been administered; epileptic activity *per se* is not a recognized feature of enflurane anaesthesia *(Ch. 8, A & S)*.
e **True** This is a late sign of cerebral damage.

(Ch. 22, A & S; Ch. 15, BNF)
a **False** It is formulated as a powder for reconstitution, and the resultant solution is alkaline.
b **False** It may be given orally preoperatively, as prophylaxis in a patient susceptible to malignant hyperthermia.
c **True** Dantrolene interferes with calcium efflux in the muscle cell, preventing the contractile process.
d **True** Liver function tests should be checked regularly in patients receiving long-term therapy.
e **True** Its site of action is on the sarcoplasmic reticulum.

29 Propranolol
a has local anaesthetic effects.
b causes postural hypotension.
c is contraindicated in patients with paroxysmal nocturnal dyspnoea (PND) and orthopnoea.
d has a half-life of 6 h.
e is a cardioselective beta-agonist.

30 Glyceryl trinitrate causes
a reduction in pulmonary arterial pressure.

b reduction in preload.
c bronchospasm.
d headache.

e relief of angina as a result of coronary artery dilatation.

31 The following drugs are absorbed well from the alimentary tract:
a ergotamine.

b oxytocin.
c atropine.

d pentamethonium.
e adrenaline.

32 The opium poppy contains
a diamorphine.
b codeine.
c thebaine.
d methadone.
e strophanthin.

(Ch. 12, A & S)

a	**True**	This is not a characteristic of all beta-blocking agents.
b	**False**	
c	**True**	Orthopnoea and PND indicate incipient heart failure, which is an absolute contraindication to propranolol therapy.
d	**False**	The majority of beta-blockers have a half-life of 3–4 h.
e	**False**	Propranolol is neither cardioselective nor an agonist.

(Ch. 13, A & S)

a	**True**	It is predominantly a venodilator, but also causes pulmonary vasodilatation.
b	**True**	Venodilatation leads to a reduction in CVP and preload.
c	**False**	
d	**True**	This is a common side-effect, because of cerebral vasodilatation.
e	**False**	Reduction in preload leads to reduction in myocardial oxygen consumption *(Ch. 9, D)*.

(Ch. 7, A & S)

a	**False**	This drug is frequently given orally, but absorption is unpredictable and the recommended routes of administration are sublingual, rectal or by inhalation *(Ch. 4, BNF)*.
b	**False**	This is usually given intravenously *(Ch. 7, BNF)*.
c	**True**	This has antispasmodic actions and is available as oral tablets *(Ch. 1, BNF)*.
d	**False**	Pentamethonium is a highly polar compound.
e	**False**	Adrenaline is usually administered systemically.

(Ch. 10, A & S)

a	**False**	Diamorphine (di-acetylmorphine) is a semi-synthetic drug.
b	**True**	
c	**True**	Buprenorphine is a thebaine derivative.
d	**False**	Methadone is a synthetic opioid.
e	**False**	Strophanthin is an alternative name for ouabain, a cardiac glycoside *(Ch. 13, A & S)*.

33 **The following antimicrobials are active against Gram-negative bacilli:**
a nitrofurantoin.

b teicoplanin.

c benzylpenicillin.
d ciprafloxacin.
e chloramphenicol.

---

34 **Rocuronium**
a is an aminosteroid.
b has a similar molecular weight to vecuronium.
c causes a bradycardia.
d has a prolonged action in renal failure.
e undergoes partial metabolism by plasma cholinesterase.

---

35 **Diuretics may act by**
a increasing the blood supply to the kidney.

b enhancing tubular reabsorption of water by osmotic action.

c preventing tubular reabsorption of Na^+.

d inhibiting the action of aldosterone.
e inhibiting the action of carbonic anhydrase.

---

36 **The following factors favour rapid and complete gastrointestinal uptake of a drug:**
a low gastric pH.

b enhanced gastric emptying.

c high lipid-solubility of the drug.
d extensive first-pass metabolism.

e rectal administration.

(Ch. 5, BNF)

a	**True**	This is recommended for urinary tract infections, 90% of which are caused by *E. coli*.
b	**False**	This is used as an alternative to vancomycin in prophylaxis of endocarditis.
c	**False**	This is used classically against Gram-positive cocci.
d	**True**	
e	**True**	This is active against both Gram-negative and Gram-positive bacteria, but is used classically against *Haemophilus influenzae*.

(Ch. 11, A & S)

a	**True**	
b	**True**	However, its onset time is faster.
c	**False**	There is a mild vagolytic action.
d	**True**	Rocuronium undergoes renal excretion.
e	**False**	Mivacurium undergoes metabolism in this way.

(Ch. 13, A & S)

a	**False**	Although dopamine increases urine output as a result of renal artery dilatation, it is not usually classified as a diuretic.
b	**False**	Osmotic diuretics (e.g. mannitol) restrict reabsorption of water from the tubules because of high osmolality.
c	**True**	Diuretics of high potency (e.g. frusemide) inhibit sodium reabsorption in the proximal tubule and loop of Henle. Low potency diuretics (e.g. acetazolamide) act mainly on the distal tubule.
d	**True**	Spironolactone is an aldosterone antagonist.
e	**True**	Thiazide diuretics act here, but their main action is on the distal tubule.

(Ch. 7, A & S)

a	**False**	Little gastric absorption occurs because the surface area is low in comparison with the small intestine. No significant benefit is gained from alterations in gastric pH.
b	**True**	This is the most important factor, as most absorption takes place in the small intestine.
c	**True**	This is important for diffusion to take place across the mucosa.
d	**False**	Extensive first-pass metabolism reduces the bioavailability of the drug.
e	**True**	Absorption takes place via both systemic and portal venous systems.

37 Frusemide

a   may cause deafness.

b   has a duration of action of 10 h when given orally.
c   may lead to decreased plasma potassium concentration.
d   produces a diuresis which is proportional to glomerular filtration rate (GFR).
e   raises plasma uric acid concentrations.

---

38 The following are true:

a   Tetracyclines cause discolouration and hypoplasia of growing teeth.
b   Chloramphenicol is a bacteriostatic antibiotic.

c   Aminoglycosides may prolong neuromuscular block.

d   Probenecid prevents tubular secretion of cephalosporins and promotes higher blood concentrations of the antibacterial agent.
e   Phenytoin prolongs the effect of thiopentone.

---

39 Gentamicin

a   is absorbed well from gastric mucosa.

b   is an aminoglycoside.

c   causes VIIIth nerve injury.

d   may cause neuromuscular blockade.

e   may cause renal damage.

---

40 There is a decreased likelihood of placental transfer of a drug if it

a   is lipid-insoluble.

b   has a molecular weight greater than 600.

c   is metabolized slowly.

d   is highly ionized.
e   is administered in small doses.

(Ch. 13, A & S)

a	**True**	Large doses of frusemide given rapidly may cause transient deafness.
b	**False**	The duration of action of oral frusemide is normally 4–6 h.
c	**True**	Frusemide enhances potassium excretion in the kidney.
d	**False**	The diuresis produced by frusemide is inversely related to GFR. Frusemide is effective at low glomerular filtration rates.
e	**True**	It shares this property with bumetanide, ethacrynic acid and the thiazide diuretics.

(Ch. 5, BNF)

a	**True**	They are contraindicated where new bone is being laid down, such as in children.
b	**True**	This is described as bacteriostatic in low doses but bactericidal in larger doses.
c	**True**	These act as antagonists at the neuromuscular junction, in a fashion similar to curare. Potentiation of curare-like drugs has been reported only with large doses of neomycin given intraperitoneally *(Ch. 4, A & S)*.
d	**True**	This is excreted preferentially, rather than beta-lactam antibiotics. This prolongs the effect of the antibiotics.
e	**False**	Liver enzyme induction may decrease the effect.

(Ch. 2, D)

a	**False**	In common with other aminoglycosides, it is not absorbed and must be given parenterally.
b	**True**	Other aminoglycosides include streptomycin, kanamycin, tobramycin, netilmicin, amikacin and neomycin.
c	**True**	Ototoxicity and nephrotoxicity are side-effects shared by all of these agents.
d	**True**	This is a theoretical interaction which seems to be unimportant clinically.
e	**True**	The combination of frusemide and aminoglycoside antibiotics is particularly nephrotoxic.

(Ch. 5, A & S)

a	**True**	Drugs must be soluble in lipid membranes to cross the placenta.
b	**True**	Compounds of small molecular weight cross the placental barrier more readily.
c	**False**	A slowly metabolized drug has higher blood concentrations and a greater diffusion gradient for a longer period than one which is metabolized rapidly.
d	**True**	Highly ionized drugs are less lipid-soluble.
e	**False**	Placental transfer depends more upon plasma concentration and pK_a of the drug than dose.

41   Sevoflurane
   a   contains seven fluoride ions.
   b   is less soluble than nitrous oxide.
   c   is incompatible with soda lime.
   d   is metabolized to a similar extent to enflurane.
   e   is non-flammable in oxygen.

42   Histamine causes
   a   an increase in arterial pressure.

   b   increased gastrointestinal motility.
   c   bronchoconstriction.
   d   pupillary dilation.
   e   stimulation of the CNS.

43   Sulphonylureas
   a   displace insulin from beta cells in the pancreas.
   b   can be used in the treatment of ketosis.

   c   are highly protein-bound.
   d   include metoclopramide within the group.

   e   may lead to acidosis.

44   The following pairs comprise an agonist and a competitive antagonist:
   a   morphine and naloxone.
   b   histamine and promethazine.

   c   phenobarbitone and doxapram.

   d   acetylcholine and gallamine.
   e   hexamethonium and methoxamine.

(Ch. 8, A & S)

a	**True**	Its formula is $CH(CF_3)_2OCH_2F$.
b	**False**	Its blood/gas partition coefficient is 0.6.
c	**False**	Hydrolysis under normal conditions is minimal.
d	**True**	2–3% is metabolized, with release of fluorine.
e	**False**	

(Ch. 4, A & S)

a	**False**	It produces peripheral vasodilatation and systemic hypotension.
b	**True**	Because of smooth muscle contraction.
c	**True**	Anatomical dead space is decreased.
d	**False**	Histamine has no effect upon pupillary diameter.
e	**False**	Although histamine receptors do exist in the CNS.

(Ch. 8, D)

a	**True**	
b	**False**	They are inappropriate for the treatment of ketosis or ketoacidosis.
c	**True**	This accounts for their long half-life.
d	**False**	Chlorpropamide is an example of the sulphonylureas – metoclopramide is a dopamine antagonist.
e	**False**	Lactic acidosis may occur with the biguanides.

(Ch. 7, A & S)

a	**True**	
b	**True**	Promethazine is a phenothiazine, and possesses potent H-receptor blocking actions *(Ch. 10, A & S)*.
c	**False**	Doxapram is an analeptic agent, and causes CNS stimulation. It may reverse effects of phenobarbitone, but in a non-competitive manner *(Ch. 10, A & S)*.
d	**True**	
e	**False**	Methoxamine is a direct-acting α-agonist; hexamethonium is a ganglion-blocking drug.

45 **The following drugs have adverse effects on bone marrow:**
a nitrous oxide in prolonged administration.

b phenylbutazone.

c phenytoin.

d phenobarbitone.
e paracetamol.

46 **The initial actions of intravenous mannitol include**
a increased blood viscosity.

b increased haematocrit.

c expansion of the blood volume.
d haemolysis.

e reduction of extracellular volume.

47 **The following antibiotics may be administered orally:**
a cefotaxime.

b kanamycin.

c vancomycin.

d ticarcillin.

e flucloxacillin.

48 **Jaundice has been associated with administration of the following:**
a diethyl ether.
b isoflurane.

c halothane.

d enflurane.

e argon.

a **True** Caused by inhibition of methionine synthetase activity *(Ch. 8, A & S)*.
b **True** This may cause agranulocytosis and aplastic anaemia *(Ch. 10, BNF)*.
c **True** This has been reported, but the commonest problem is megaloblastic anaemia, because of folate deficiency *(Ch. 4, BNF)*.
d **False**
e **False** Although methionine depletion has been reported, there was no depression of bone marrow function *(Ch. 19, D)*.

(Ch. 28, A & S)

a **False** Dilution of intravascular fluid causes a decrease in blood viscosity.
b **False** Initially, water is drawn from the intracellular to the extracellular space, thereby raising plasma volume and reducing haematocrit.
c **True** See **b** above.
d **False** The hyperosmolarity of mannitol results in red cell shrinkage, not haemolysis.
e **True** See **b** above.

(Ch. 2, D; Ch. 5, BNF)

a **False** This is a third-generation cephalosporin, which is administered only by intramuscular or i.v. injection.
b **False** This is an aminoglycoside, which is inactive after oral administration.
c **True** Although this is available orally, parenteral administration is the method of choice. It is employed frequently for the prophylaxis of bacterial endocarditis preoperatively.
d **False** This is the successor to carbenicillin. It is used parenterally against *Pseudomonas* infections.
e **True** This is the oral antistaphylococcal drug of choice.

(Ch. 8, A & S)

a **True**
b **False** Jaundice has not been reported. Isoflurane undergoes minimal hepatic metabolism.
c **True** Jaundice may be associated with the use of halothane (especially after repeated exposure within a short space of time).
d **True** Although rarer than with halothane, liver failure and jaundice have been reported following enflurane administration.
e **False** Argon is an inert gas.

(Ch. 13, A & S)

49 The following drugs may act on the chemoreceptor trigger zone (CTZ):

a digoxin.

b droperidol.

c morphine.

d metoclopramide.

e hyoscine.

---

50 The following agents decrease arterial pressure by a central action:
a hexamethonium.
b propranolol.
c prazosin.
d clonidine.
e tubocurarine.

---

51 Methaemoglobinaemia may follow administration of
a sodium citrate.
b methylene blue.

c procaine.
d prilocaine.

e cinchocaine.

---

52 Heparin
a is a synthetic acid.
b is found in mast cells.

c is released during anaphylactic shock.
d is an antiplasmin.

e causes thrombocytopenia.

(Ch. 13, A & S)

a **False**   This commonly causes loss of appetite, nausea and vomiting, but not due to an effect upon the CTZ.
b **True**   This is a specific dopamine antagonist, which acts on the CTZ and is a powerful antiemetic.
c **True**   This depresses the CNS generally, but stimulates the CTZ and the Edinger–Westphal nucleus (miosis) *(Ch. 10, A & S)*.
d **True**   This has peripheral actions which enhance gastric emptying, and a specific dopamine antagonistic effect on the CTZ.
e **False**   This is a CNS depressant and an anticholinergic; it has antiemetic actions but no direct effect upon the CTZ.

(Ch. 36, A & S)

a **False**   This is a ganglion blocker.
b **False**   This agent possesses negative inotropic properties.
c **False**   Prazosin is an alpha$_1$-blocker *(Ch. 12, A & S)*.
d **True**   Clonidine is an α_2-agonist *(Ch. 2, BNF)*.
e **False**   This reduces arterial pressure by a combination of ganglion blockade and histamine release.

---

a **False**
b **False**   This is the agent of choice for treatment of methaemoglobinaemia.
c **False**
d **True**   This produces *o*-toluidine, leading to methaemoglobinaemia, but only if doses considerably in excess of 600 mg are administered *(Ch. 14, A & S)*.
e **False**

(Ch. 11, D)

a **False**   Heparin is a complex polysaccharide.
b **True**   It is one of the agents released in anaphylactic shock from the degranulation of the mast cell in response to stimulation of reaginic antibodies.
c **True**   See **b** above.
d **False**   Heparin is not an antiplasmin. It accelerates the action of antithrombin III.
e **True**

53 The following are positive inotropes:

a isoprenaline.

b aminophylline.

c fenfluramine.
d methoxamine.
e enalapril.

---

54 Hypoglycaemia occurs after administration of

a glucagon.

b tolbutamide.
c diazoxide.
d hydrocortisone.

e propranolol.

---

55 The following are beta-blockers:

a diltiazem.
b oxprenolol.

c chlorpromazine.
d salbutamol.
e metoprolol.

---

56 Bronchodilation is produced by

a atropine.

b methohexitone.
c ephedrine.

d vecuronium.
e oxprenolol.

(Ch. 12, A & S)

a	**True**	This is a β-agonist which stimulates both the cardiac $beta_1$- and bronchial $beta_2$-receptors.
b	**True**	This stimulates cAMP; it is a positive chronotrope and inotrope, with a dominant action on $beta_2$-receptors.
c	**False**	Fenfluramine is an appetite suppressant.
d	**False**	Methoxamine is an $alpha_1$-adrenoceptor agonist.
e	**False**	Enalapril is an angiotensin-converting enzyme inhibitor.

(Ch. 8, D)

a	**False**	This is produced by the alpha cells of the pancreas, and increases blood glucose concentration.
b	**True**	This is a suphonylurea oral hypoglycaemic agent.
c	**False**	This is a vasodilator which causes hyperglycaemia *(Ch. 2, BNF)*.
d	**False**	This enhances gluconeogenesis and glycogenolysis, and therefore causes hyperglycaemia.
e	**True**	This may block the response to hyperglycaemia. Although propranolol is not contraindicated absolutely in diabetics, a cardioselective beta-blocker is preferable *(Ch. 2, BNF)*.

(Ch. 12, A & S)

a	**False**	This is a calcium-channel blocker.
b	**True**	This is a beta-blocking agent with partial agonist activity and a membrane-stabilizing effect.
c	**False**	This has alpha-adrenergic blocking actions but no beta-effects.
d	**False**	This is a $β_2$-agonist.
e	**True**	This is cardioselective and has a membrane-stabilizing effect.

(Ch. 12, A & S)

a	**True**	Bronchoconstriction is a muscarinic effect of acetylcholine, and is antagonized by atropine.
b	**False**	
c	**True**	Ephedrine is a directly and indirectly acting sympathomimetic agent.
d	**False**	Vecuronium can only occasionally cause release of histamine.
e	**False**	Oxprenolol is a beta-adrenergic blocking drug which is not cardioselective; consequently, it may cause bronchoconstriction.

57 **Drugs whose actions are reduced in the presence of hepatic enzyme induction include**
a fentanyl.
b phenobarbitone.

c diazepam.
d halothane.

e warfarin.

---

58 **Thrombophlebitis may follow i.v. administration of**
a midazolam.
b propofol.

c thiopentone.

d diazepam.

e atracurium.

---

59 **Duration of action of the barbiturates is decreased by**
a substitution of sulphur for oxygen in the 2 position.

b methylation in the 1 or 3 position.

c formation of sodium salts.

d branching of carbon chains in the 5 position.

e desaturation of carbon chains.

---

60 **The clearance of a drug**
a is equal to the liver blood flow.

b is the same for all drugs with first-order kinetics.
c may be calculated from the area under the plasma concentration–time curve (AUC).
d is equal to the infusion rate at steady state.
e has the units of reciprocal time.

(Ch. 7, A & S)

a **False** The action of fentanyl is terminated by redistribution.
b **True** Phenobarbitone is long-acting, and liver metabolism is responsible for terminating its action. Phenobarbitone causes enzyme induction.
c **False** Diazepam has a pharmacologically active metabolite.
d **False** Halothane metabolites may be responsible for toxicity. Metabolites are more likely in the presence of enzyme induction.
e **True** The dose may require frequent adjustment in the presence of an enzyme-inducing drug.

(Ch. 23, A & S)

a **False**
b **False** This is remarkably devoid of venous thrombotic sequelae or perivascular reactions, but pain on injection is common.
c **True** Although uncommon, this does occur. In addition, extravascular injection may result in tissue necrosis.
d **True** Venous sequelae are very common after i.v. diazepam unless the lipid formulation (Diazemuls) is used.
e **False** No association has been demonstrated between venous thrombosis and use of atracurium.

(Ch. 9, A & S)

a **True** This enhances lipid-solubility and confers rapidity of onset, with short duration of action.
b **True** Methylation, particularly in the 1 position, produces a rapid-acting drug with a short duration of action – but convulsive activity is more likely.
c **False** All the intravenous barbiturates are formulated as sodium salts, in order to improve solubility.
d **True** Alterations in the 5 position affect potency. Increase in potency and decrease in duration of action are produced by increasing the length of the side chains or by branching of the side chains.
e **True** Double bonds in the side chains are metabolized more easily.

(Ch. 7, A & S)

a **False** Clearance is the sum of all clearances including liver, renal, pulmonary, etc.
b **False**
c **True** In a two-compartment model, clearance = dose/AUC.
d **False** At steady state, clearance = infusion rate/plasma concentration.
e **False** The units are volume of plasma/time.

61 **The following are available in a fat emulsion:**
  a propofol.

  b eltanolone.
  c ketamine.
  d diazepam.
  e midazolam.

62 **Hartmann's solution contains**
  a sodium 112 mmol/l.
  b chloride 131 mmol/l.
  c bicarbonate 29 mmol/l.

  d calcium 2.4 mmol/l.

  e potassium 1.5 mmol/l.

63 **Oxprenolol**
  a may cause increased airway resistance.

  b decreases peripheral blood flow.
  c may cause hypoglycaemia.

  d may be used to treat symptoms of thyrotoxicosis.

  e has a bioavailability of less than 50%.

64 **Lignocaine**
  a may exhibit tachyphylaxis if used as an epidural infusion.
  b does not cross the placenta.
  c is lipid-soluble as a base but water-soluble as the hydrochloride.

  d does not depress smooth muscle.

  e is anticonvulsant.

(Ch. 9, A & S)

a	**True**	This is prepared as an emulsion in 10% Intralipid in a concentration of 10 mg/ml.
b	**True**	This is 5β-pregnanolone in 10% Intralipid.
c	**False**	This is available in aqueous acidic solution.
d	**True**	Diazemuls is diazepam 5 mg/ml in Intralipid.
e	**False**	This is a water-soluble benzodiazepine *(Ch. 10, A & S)*.

(Appendix VId, A & S)

a	**False**	It contains 131 mmol/l of sodium.
b	**False**	It contains 112 mmol/l of chloride.
c	**False**	It contains 29 mmol/l of lactate, which is converted to bicarbonate by the liver. Bicarbonate is precipitated in the presence of calcium.
d	**True**	This approximates to the normal plasma concentration of calcium.
e	**False**	It contains 5 mmol/l of potassium.

(Ch. 12, A & S)

a	**True**	Beta$_2$-blockade causes bronchiolar constriction and an increase in airway resistance.
b	**True**	This results from unopposed alpha-receptor stimulation.
c	**False**	It may aggravate diabetes mellitus by provoking hyperglycaemia. In addition, the response to hypoglycaemia may be impaired.
d	**True**	Beta-blockers are effective in the treatment of the symptoms of thyrotoxicosis, but do not influence thyrotoxicosis.
e	**True**	There is significant first-pass metabolism, but this is offset by the production of active metabolites.

(Ch. 14, A & S)

a	**True**	All local anaesthetics have a tendency to exhibit tachyphylaxis.
b	**False**	All local anaesthetic agents cross the placenta.
c	**True**	It is presented as the hydrochloride because the basic form is lipid-soluble.
d	**True**	It does not have any direct vasoconstrictor or vasodilator action.
e	**True**	Although toxic manifestations include convulsions, these are caused by cortical depression; inherently, it is a CNS depressant.

65 Atropine
a exhibits more cardiac effects than hyoscine.
b is more sedative than hyoscine.
c is a more effective antisialogogue than glycopyrrolate.

d causes hyperpyrexia in overdosage.

e reduces physiological dead space.

66 Dopamine antagonists
a cause extrapyramidal side-effects.

b may be used as antiemetics.

c may increase gastric emptying.

d cause tachycardia.

e may cause peripheral vasoconstriction.

67 Atracurium
a is metabolized solely by Hofmann degradation.

b is metabolized to laudanosine.

c causes neuromuscular block which is prolonged by hypothermia.

d causes neuromuscular block which is prolonged by low pH.
e does not release histamine.

68 Alfentanil
a is cardiodepressant.
b is more potent than fentanyl.

c is more lipid-soluble than fentanyl.
d has a shorter elimination half-life than fentanyl.

e is antagonized by naloxone.

(Ch. 12, A & S)

a **True**
b **False** Hyoscine is more sedative, especially in the elderly subject.
c **False** Glycopyrronium bromide is a quaternary amine with antisialogogue properties which are more pronounced than those of atropine.
d **True** The use of atropine is contraindicated in the presence of pyrexia, especially in children.
e **False** Physiological dead space is increased by 20%.

(Ch. 10, A & S)

a **True** Agents such as the phenothiazines and butyrophenones are notable for extrapyramidal side-effects.
b **True** Dopamine antagonists have a powerful action on the CTZ which is physiologically outwith the blood–brain barrier.
c **True** Domperidone and metoclopramide are dopamine antagonists which increase the rate of gastric emptying and the tone of the lower oesophageal sphincter.
d **False** Dopamine antagonists do not cause tachycardia *per se*. However, some dopamine antagonists (e.g. chlorpromazine) also effect alpha-receptor blockade and this may lead to a tachycardia secondary to vasodilatation.
e **False** Some dopamine antagonists may cause vasodilatation by alpha-adrenergic blocking actions.

(Ch. 11, A & S)

a **False** It is metabolized by ester hydrolysis in addition to Hofmann degradation.
b **True** This is one of the breakdown products of atracurium. However, not all of an administered dose is converted to this compound.
c **True** Breakdown of atracurium is slower in the presence of hypothermia and is accelerated by hyperthermia.
d **True** Breakdown is decreased in an acid environment.
e **False** Histamine release occurs to an extent of a third that of curare.

(Ch. 10, A & S)

a **False** Alfentanil is not cardiodepressant *per se*.
b **False** It has a much more rapid onset than other opioids but is less potent (ratio = 4:1) than fentanyl.
c **False** It is less lipid-soluble.
d **True** The elimination half-life of fentanyl is 4 h, whereas that of alfentanil is 1.5 h. However, clearance of fentanyl is three times that of alfentanil.
e **True** Naloxone antagonizes the actions of all μ-receptor agonists.

69 Diamorphine

a is more potent than morphine.
b cannot be used in terminal care because of tolerance.

c causes more euphoria than morphine.
d is a potent cough suppressant.
e is a constituent of opium.

70 Vecuronium

a causes bradycardia.

b has a steroid structure.
c is contraindicated in the presence of renal failure.
d does not release histamine.
e contains two quaternary nitrogen groups.

71 Human albumin solution (HAS)

a is stored at room temperature.
b is prepared from pooled blood and may transmit hepatitis B.
c contains not less than 40 g/l of protein.
d is used to treat disseminated intravascular coagulation (DIC).
e contains approximately 150 mmol/l of sodium.

72 Mivacurium

a is an aminosteroid relaxant.
b is metabolized by cholinesterase.
c does not release histamine.
d does not require reversal with anticholinesterase.

e is presented as a powder.

73 The action of suxamethonium is prolonged by

a lignocaine.
b propofol.
c ecothiopate.

d neostigmine.
e organophosphate insecticides

(Ch. 10, A & S)

a **True** Diamorphine is two to three times more potent than morphine.
b **False** Tolerance does occur, but this is not usually a consideration in terminal care as the dose is increased if necessary.
c **True**
d **True** All opioids are effective antitussive agents.
e **False** Diamorphine is a condensation product of acetic acid and morphine. It is not a constituent of opium.

(Ch. 11, A & S)

a **False** Vecuronium has no actions on the heart. Bradycardia may occur intraoperatively as a result of surgical manipulation.
b **True** However, it possesses no hormonal activity.
c **False** It is metabolized by the liver to inactive metabolites.
d **True**
e **False** However, the second tertiary nitrogen is capable of attracting a hydrogen ion in vivo.

(Ch. 6, and Appendix VId, A & S)

a **True** It has a 3-year shelf-life at room temperature.
b **False** It is heat-treated and this inactivates the hepatitis virus.
c **True** It contains approximately 45 g/l of protein.
d **False** It is low in coagulation factors.
e **True**

(Ch. 11, A & S)

a **False** It is a benzylisoquinolinium ester.
b **True** The rate of metabolism is 70–88% that of suxamethonium.
c **False** This occurs with doses of $> 2 \times ED_{95}$.
d **True** But neuromuscular function should be monitored to ensure reversal.
e **False**

(Ch. 11, A & S)

a **False**
b **False**
c **True** This is an anticholinesterase, used as eye-drops but with systemic activity.
d **True** This is an anticholinesterase.
e **True** Organophosphorus anticholinesterases used in chemical warfare and insecticides have actions which are not easily reversible *(Ch. 19, D)*.

74 Ropivacaine
  a is an ester-linked local anaesthetic.
  b has a greater potency than bupivacaine.
  c has a longer duration of action than bupivacaine.
  d is 20% less protein-bound than bupivacaine.
  e contains preservative.

75 Beta-blocking drugs
  a become less beta-selective with increasing dosage.

  b are contraindicated in heart failure.

  c are classified as Vaughan Williams group III.

  d are indicated in the treatment of supraventricular tachycardia (SVT).
  e may cause peripheral vasoconstriction.

76 Digitalis is employed commonly for the treatment of
  a atrial flutter.
  b idioventricular rhythm.

  c ventricular tachycardia.
  d cardiac tamponade.
  e 2:1 atrioventricular (AV) block.

77 Cocaine
  a causes pupillary constriction.

  b is a drug of dependence.

  c is a synthetic drug.
  d is employed as a 10% solution.
  e is an ester.

(Ch. 14, A & S)

a **False** It has an amide link.
b **False** It is less potent.
c **False** Its duration is similar.
d **False** Protein binding is similar.
e **False** Preservative-free preparations only may be used in the extradural space.

(Ch. 12, A & S)

a **True** As with all agents acting on the sympathetic nervous system, beta-blocking drugs become less specific with increasing dosage.
b **True** Beta-blocking drugs worsen heart failure by decreasing myocardial contractility.
c **False** Beta-blocking drugs comprise group II of the Vaughan Williams classification of anti-arrhythmic drugs. Group III comprises those drugs delaying repolarization, such as amiodarone.
d **True** They are very effective in the treatment of SVT *(Ch. 2, BNF)*.
e **True** However, the mechanism causing this is unclear *(Ch. 2, BNF)*.

(Ch. 13, A & S; Ch. 3, D)

a **True** It is used to control the ventricular rate.
b **False** A pacemaker is the most appropriate therapy for this condition.
c **False** It is indicated for supraventricular arrhythmias.
d **False**
e **False** It depresses AV conduction and therefore increases the block.

(Ch. 14, A & S)

a **False** It has sympathomimetic properties and causes pupillary dilation.
b **True** It is a controlled drug governed by Schedule 2 of the Misuse of Drugs Regulations *(BNF)*.
c **False** It is the alkaloid of the coca plant.
d **False** Cocaine is available as a 1–4% solution.
e **True** It is a benzoic acid ester.

78 Bupivacaine

    a has a duration of action longer than that of lignocaine.

    b is contraindicated in intravenous regional anaesthesia (IVRA).

    c is metabolized mainly by the liver.

    d is more cardiotoxic than lignocaine.

    e is available in solutions containing 1:100 000 adrenaline.

---

79 The following drugs undergo significant metabolism in the liver:
    a pethidine.
    b lignocaine.
    c halothane.

    d noradrenaline.

    e chlorpromazine.

---

80 The following produce marked systemic analgesia:
    a droperidol.
    b perphenazine.
    c promethazine.
    d nalbuphine.
    e fentanyl.

---

81 Ketorolac
    a is contraindicated during pregnancy.
    b may be admininstered i.m.
    c stimulates the CTZ.
    d inhibits the activity of cyclo-oxygenase.
    e is nephrotoxic.

(Ch. 14, A & S)

a **True** It has a duration of action two to four times greater than that of lignocaine.

b **True** It is contraindicated in IVRA because of marked cardiovascular depression, which can occur after bolus intravenous injections.

c **True** Bupivacaine is an amide and is metabolized mainly by the liver.

d **True** The toxic dose is 2 mg/kg and bupivacaine produces cardiotoxicity before CNS depression.

e **False** Preparations of bupivacaine are available with 1:200 000 or 1:400 000 adrenaline (50 μg/ml and 25 μg/ml respectively).

(Ch. 7, A & S)

a **True** It is demethylated in the liver.

b **True** This is an amide and undergoes metabolism in the liver.

c **True** Approximately 20% of an inhaled dose of halothane undergoes metabolism in the liver by various mechanisms, including oxidation and reduction *(Ch. 8, A & S)*.

d **False** It is metabolized mainly at the nerve terminals by catechol-*o*-methyl transferase. Only a small proportion of noradrenaline secreted by nerve terminals enters the circulation and is metabolized by the liver.

e **True** It undergoes a phase I reaction in the liver, resulting in pharmacologically active metabolites. It may cause jaundice of a cholestatic type.

(Ch. 10, A & S)

a **False** This is a butyrophenone.

b **False** This is a phenothiazine.

c **False** This is a phenothiazine.

d **True** This is a μ-antagonist but a κ-agonist.

e **True** This is a synthetic opioid analgesic derived from pethidine.

(Ch. 15, BNF)

a **True** NSAIDs are contraindicated during pregnancy.

b **True**

c **False** NSAIDs have no action here.

d **True** This is its main mechanism of action.

e **True** Its use has been limited by this effect.

82 **The following drugs are associated with spontaneous muscle movements:**
a propofol.

b diazepam.
c haloperidol.

d perphenazine.
e suxamethonium.

83 **Morphine**
a increases intrabiliary pressure.
b reduces urine output.
c releases histamine.
d is associated with neutropenia in prolonged use.

e causes increased baroreceptor traffic.

84 **The action of non-depolarizing neuromuscular blocking drugs is influenced by**
a atypical cholinesterase.

b gentamicin.

c plasma proteins.

d hyponatraemia.
e hypothermia.

85 **Thiazide diuretics may produce**
a hyponatraemia.
b hypokalaemic alkalosis.
c hyperuricaemia.
d hyperchloraemia.
e weight loss.

(Ch. 9, A & S)

a **True** Tonic and clonic movements may occur on induction, but are reduced by rapid administration.
b **False** This decreases muscle tone.
c **True** This is a dopamine antagonist and causes extrapyramidal side-effects.
d **True** This is a phenothiazine.
e **True** This results from fasciculations, which are characteristic of depolarizing block.

(Ch. 10, A & S)

a **True**
b **True** It stimulates release of antidiuretic hormone (ADH).
c **True** It acts directly on mast cells to release histamine.
d **False** This occurs with N_2O, not morphine. However, morphine reduces reticuloendothelial system activity and phagocytosis by white blood cells.
e **False** It may cause hypotension as a result of vasodilatation secondary to central depression. Decreased baroreceptor activity ensues.

(Ch. 11, A & S)

a **False** Atypical cholinesterase affects the metabolism of suxamethonium.
b **True** This effect was described first with intraperitoneal neomycin, another aminoglycoside.
c **True** Non-depolarizing neuromuscular blockers are bound to plasma proteins, and alterations in the concentrations of free drugs affect bioavailability.
d **False** Hyponatraemia has no influence.
e **True** Hypothermia usually prolongs the action of non-depolarizing neuromuscular blockers.

(Ch. 13, A & S)

a **False** Water and sodium are excreted together.
b **True** Potassium loss occurs, with secondary metabolic alkalosis.
c **True** This is caused by interference with uric acid excretion.
d **False** Hypochloraemia is more common.
e **True** Caused by water loss.

86 **The following drugs are calcium-channel blockers:**
a verapamil.

b enalapril.
c propranolol.
d nifedipine.
e hydralazine.

87 **The following impurities may occur in nitrous oxide:**
a nitrogen.
b nitric oxide.

c nitroglycerine.

d nitrogen dioxide.
e metal oxides.

88 **Sucralfate**
a contains aluminium.
b is an H_2-receptor antagonist.
c inhibits pepsin activity.
d binds to mucoprotein.
e may potentiate opioid sedation.

89 **The actions of benzodiazepines**
a result from inhibition of GABA receptors.

b include profound retrograde amnesia.
c relieve acute anxiety.
d may result in respiratory depression.
e mostly result from active metabolites.

90 **The pupil is dilated by instillation of the following drugs into the conjunctival sac:**
a ephedrine.
b timolol.

c homatropine.
d cocaine.
e chloramphenicol.

(Ch. 13, A & S)

a	**True**	This was the first commercially available calcium-channel blocking drug.
b	**False**	This is an angiotensin-converting enzyme inhibitor.
c	**False**	This is a beta-adrenoceptor blocker.
d	**True**	
e	**False**	This is a direct-acting vasodilator.

(Ch. 8, A & S)

a	**True**	Nitrogen is present in the manufacture of nitrous oxide.
b	**True**	Nitric oxide occurs as an impurity during manufacture and is removed by 'scrubbing' with water, with which it forms nitrous acid.
c	**False**	Nitroglycerine is formed by heating glycerine with concentrated nitric acid. It is not a by-product of manufacture of nitrous oxide.
d	**True**	This is removed by 'scrubbing' with water to form nitric acid.
e	**False**	Metal oxides are not produced from the decomposition of ammonium nitrate (NH_4NO_3).

(Ch. 13, A & S)

a	**True**	It is aluminium hydroxide and sulphated sucrose.
b	**False**	
c	**True**	
d	**True**	It exerts its gastric protective effect in this way.
e	**False**	It is largely unabsorbed.

(Ch. 10, A & S)

a	**False**	The actions of the inhibitory transmitter, GABA, are facilitated by benzodiazepines.
b	**False**	Anterograde amnesia only occurs.
c	**True**	This action renders the group useful for premedication.
d	**True**	Particularly on i.v. administration.
e	**False**	Diazepam has an active metabolite but other members of the group do not.

(Ch. 11, BNF)

a	**True**	Ephedrine has sympathomimetic actions.
b	**False**	Timolol is a beta-blocker used in the treatment of glaucoma; it causes pupillary constriction.
c	**True**	Homatropine has a shorter duration of action than atropine.
d	**True**	It possesses sympathomimetic actions.
e	**False**	

91 Lithium
 a inhibits release of noradrenaline.
 b potentiates neuromuscular block.

 c is excreted by the renal tubules.
 d has a narrow therapeutic ratio.
 e is more toxic in the presence of hypernatraemia.

92 Flumazenil
 a antagonizes the actions of lorazepam.
 b may be administered orally.
 c does not reverse the amnesic actions of benzodiazepines.
 d undergoes rapid metabolism in the liver.

 e prevents the benzodiazepine withdrawal syndrome.

93 Dantrolene
 a stimulates respiration.
 b is a muscle relaxant.

 c is the drug of choice for the treatment of malignant hyperthermia.
 d is a good analgesic.
 e antagonizes benzodiazepines.

94 Adrenaline
 a increases pulmonary ventilation.

 b is excreted as indole acetic acid.

 c dilates the pupil.
 d stimulates alpha-adrenoreceptors.
 e causes diastolic hypotension.

(Ch. 29, A & S)

a	**True**	Lithium is used in the treatment of manic states.
b	**True**	It substitutes for sodium ions. Both depolarizing and non-depolarizing blockers may be potentiated.
c	**True**	
d	**True**	Plasma concentrations should be monitored.
e	**False**	Lithium toxicity is exacerbated by sodium depletion.

(Ch. 10, A & S)

a	**True**	Flumazenil is a benzodiazepine antagonist.
b	**False**	It must be administered by i.v. bolus injection or i.v. infusion.
c	**False**	All central actions of benzodiazepines are antagonized.
d	**True**	Its elimination half-life is less than 1 h. Sedation and amnesia caused by long-acting benzodiazepines may return.
e	**False**	It may induce withdrawal symptoms after long-term use of benzodiazepines.

(Ch. 22, A & S)

a	**False**	It does not stimulate respiration.
b	**True**	It is a direct-acting muscle relaxant rather than a neuromuscular blocker.
c	**True**	It should be used early and in appropriate dosage.
d	**False**	It has no analgesic activity.
e	**False**	The specific benzodiazepine antagonist is flumazenil.

(Ch. 12, A & S)

a	**True**	Tachypnoea is a frequent accompaniment to sympathetic stimulation.
b	**False**	Indole acetic acid is the metabolic product of 5-hydroxyindole acetic acid and 5-hydroxytryptamine. Adrenaline is excreted in the urine as 3-methoxy-4-hydroxymandelic acid.
c	**True**	
d	**True**	It stimulates both alpha- and beta-receptors.
e	**False**	In general, adrenaline causes an increase in both peripheral resistance and cardiac output and results in hypertension. Diastolic pressure is affected less, and pulse pressure is increased.

95 Sulphonylureas

a may cause lactic acidosis.

b are useful in maturity-onset diabetes.

c may produce reactive hypoglycaemia.

d are useful in post-pancreatectomy patients.

e may cause nausea and vomiting.

---

96 Promethazine

a is an antihistamine.

b has anticholinergic actions.
c is less sedative than chlorpromazine.
d causes anterograde amnesia.
e may precipitate acute porphyria.

---

97 Properties of halothane include

a chemical structure of C_2HF_3BrCl.
b bronchoconstriction.
c MAC of 0.75.
d good analgesia at subanaesthetic concentrations.
e increase in CSF pressure.

---

98 Naloxone antagonizes the respiratory depression caused by

a enflurane.
b buprenorphine.

c pentazocine.
d phenazocine.
e barbiturates.

(Ch. 8, D)

a	**False**	This is a complication of treatment with biguanides but not sulphonylureas.
b	**True**	Maturity-onset diabetes is commonly treated with sulphonylureas.
c	**True**	Sulphonylureas may lead to hypoglycaemia occurring 4 or more hours after food and this may be an indication of overdose.
d	**False**	The sulphonylureas act mainly by augmenting the secretion of insulin.
e	**True**	Side-effects of sulphonylureas include gastrointestinal disturbances.

(Chs. 10 and 13, A & S)

a	**True**	Its antihistaminic actions are more marked than those of other phenothiazines.
b	**True**	It causes bronchodilation and reduces secretions.
c	**False**	It has a greater sedative effect than chlorpromazine.
d	**False**	
e	**True**	Antihistamines, with the exception of chlorpromazine and cyclizine, should be avoided in porphyria.

(Ch. 8, A & S)

a	**False**	Halothane is $CF_3CHClBr$ *(Appendix II, A & S)*.
b	**False**	It is a useful agent for the asthmatic patient.
c	**True**	*(Appendix II, A & S)*
d	**False**	Unlike nitrous oxide.
e	**True**	In common with other volatile agents.

(Ch. 10, A & S)

a	**False**	Enflurane has no effect at opioid receptors.
b	**True**	This is a partial agonist with very high affinity for µ-receptors. Very high doses of naloxone may be required, and non-specific ventilatory stimulants are preferred.
c	**True**	But pentazocine is an antagonist at µ-receptors.
d	**False**	*(Ch. 4, BNF)*.
e	**False**	The mechanism of ventilatory depression caused by barbiturates is different from that of opioids *(Ch. 9, A & S)*.

99   The following statements are true of local anaesthetics:

    a   The maximum safe dose of plain lignocaine is 3 mg/kg.

    b   The maximum safe dose of plain bupivacaine is 2 mg/kg.

    c   Amethocaine is hydrolysed by serum cholinesterase.

    d   Bupivacaine is an ester-linked drug.

    e   Etidocaine selectively blocks motor nerves.

100   The following have active metabolites:

    a   pethidine.

    b   atracurium.

    c   digoxin.

    d   lorazepam.

    e   remifentanil.

(Ch. 14, A & S)

a **True** But caution must be exercised when rapid intravascular injection is possible.
b **True** It is cardiotoxic.
c **True** It is a *para*-aminobenzoic acid derivative.
d **False** It is an amide and is metabolized in the liver.
e **True** This drug produces a more marked motor block than sensory block.

(Ch. 7, A & S)

a **True** Norpethidine may cause epilepsy.
b **True** Laudanosine toxicity has been reported.
c **False** Digoxin is excreted largely unchanged.
d **False**
e **False**

3. Medicine

1   A patient had a preoperative serum urea concentration of 10 mmol/l, and a serum creatinine concentration of 200 µmol/l. Several days after abdominal surgery, the urea concentration is 22 mmol/l and that of creatinine is 240 µmol/l; urine sodium content is 140 mmol/24 h and serum osmolality is 300 mosmol/kg. The following are true:
    a   The patient had disordered renal function preoperatively.
    b   The patient is now dehydrated.

    c   Intravenous fluids should be given.
    d   The likely diagnosis is an acute exacerbation of chronic renal failure.
    e   Measurement of creatinine clearance is indicated.

2   **Endotoxic septicaemia**
    a   is always produced by Gram-negative organisms.
    b   is usually associated with positive blood culture.

    c   is always associated with a low cardiac output.
    d   has a good prognosis.
    e   is relatively common after genitourinary surgery.

3   **In carbon monoxide poisoning the following are seen:**
    a   arrhythmias.
    b   hypotension.
    c   extensor plantar reflexes.
    d   cyanosis.
    e   cerebral oedema.

(Ch. 3 and Appendix IV, A & S)

a **True** The serum urea and creatinine concentrations were high.
b **False** The urinary sodium concentration and serum osmolality are within normal limits.
c **False** Careful clinical assessment is necessary before i.v. fluid therapy.
d **True** The serum urea concentration may increase rapidly postoperatively if chronic renal failure is present *(Ch. 40, A & S)*.
e **True** This would confirm the loss of renal function *(Ch. 6, D)*.

(Ch. 41, A & S)

a **False** Gram-positive organisms may be implicated in some cases.
b **False** Blood culture does not always yield positive results and antibiotic treatment should not be withheld.
c **False** Cardiac output may be elevated, especially in the early phase.
d **False** Mortality may be greater than 60%.
e **False** But genitourinary surgery is a common source of infection in bacteraemic shock *(Ch. 2, D)*.

(Ch. 19, D)

a **True** Ectopic beats and atrial fibrillation are common.
b **True** Heart failure and hypotension may develop rapidly.
c **True** This occurs if poisoning is severe.
d **False** Classically, a cherry red colour is evident if exposure is severe.
e **True** This contributes to eventual coma.

4 **The following are associated with haemophilia:**
  a haemarthrosis.

  b mucous membrane haemorrhages.

  c haemorrhagic rash.

  d decreased clot retraction.
  e positive Schilling test.

---

5 **The following may be used in the presence of reversible airways obstruction:**
  a metoprolol.
  b practolol.
  c pethidine.

  d helium.
  e propranolol.

---

6 **Tension pneumothorax**
  a is accompanied by deviation of the trachea to the opposite side.
  b is a risk of spinal cord surgery.
  c is accompanied by stridor.
  d results in a decreased arterial P_{O_2}.

  e is treated by tracheal intubation and positive pressure ventilation.

---

7 **The following are features of acute pericarditis:**
  a raised jugular venous pressure (JVP) which decreases during inspiration.
  b an association with uraemia.
  c an association with a viral illness.
  d retrosternal pain relieved only by morphine.
  e pericardial friction rub.

(Ch. 11, D)

a	**True**	Haemarthrosis is a well-recognized complication of haemophilia.
b	**False**	Mucous membrane haemorrhages are not a common complication of haemophilia.
c	**False**	Haemorrhagic rash is associated commonly with platelet deficiency.
d	**False**	Clot retraction is normal in haemophilia.
e	**False**	The Schilling test assesses uptake of vitamin B_{12} from the gut.

(Ch. 13, A & S)

a	**True**	In normal doses, metoprolol is a cardioselective beta-blocker.
b	**False**	Practolol is no longer available in the UK.
c	**True**	Pethidine has mild anticholinergic actions, releases less histamine than morphine and is preferable for asthmatic patients *(Ch. 10, A & S)*.
d	**True**	But there is no specific benefit in this situation.
e	**False**	Propranolol is a non-cardioselective beta-blocker.

(Ch. 31, A & S)

a	**True**	This results from positive pressure in the affected hemithorax.
b	**False**	There is no increased risk with spinal surgery *(Ch. 37, A & S)*.
c	**False**	Stridor is an indication of tracheal narrowing *(Ch. 4, D)*.
d	**True**	Because of hypoventilation of the lung on the affected side and increased shunting *(Ch. 1, A & S)*.
e	**False**	An intercostal chest drain should be inserted expeditiously.

(Ch. 3, D)

a	**False**	Venous congestion is typical of constrictive pericarditis.
b	**True**	Acute pericarditis may accompany uraemia.
c	**True**	Coxsackie B virus may be implicated.
d	**False**	Simple analgesia only is required.
e	**True**	Friction rub is characteristic of acute pericarditis.

8   **Intravenous entrainment of air is hazardous, particularly in patients with**

   a   patent ductus arteriosus (PDA).

   b   ventricular septal defect (VSD).

   c   pulmonary valve stenosis.

   d   patent foramen ovale.

   e   tricuspid incompetence.

---

9   **In respect of propranolol administration**

   a   left bundle branch block is a contraindication.

   b   hypokalaemia is a contraindication.

   c   digoxin therapy is a contraindication.

   d   history of nocturnal dyspnoea is a contraindication.

   e   administration may cause postural hypotension.

---

10   **The following may cause liver damage in acute overdose:**

   a   paracetamol.

   b   aspirin.
   c   paraquat.

   d   amitriptyline.

   e   halothane.

(Ch. 3, D)

a **False** Entrained air is unlikely to reach the systemic circulation, because the shunt is usually from left to right unless Eisenmenger's syndrome supervenes.
b **True** With a ventricular septal defect, right-to-left shunting occurs in the presence of systemic hypotension and/or pulmonary hypertension.
c **False** But an associated ventricular septal defect may be more dangerous in the presence of pulmonary valve stenosis.
d **True** Right-to-left shunting of blood may occur in the presence of pulmonary hypertension.
e **False** This occurs secondary to right ventricular dilatation.

(Ch. 12, A & S; Ch. 3, D)

a **True** Left bundle branch block may progress occasionally to complete heart block and idioventricular rhythm. Propranolol may produce bradycardia and exacerbate this tendency.
b **False** Hypokalaemia should be corrected but is not a contraindication to propranolol therapy.
c **False** Although there is a theoretical possibility of complete heart block with digoxin, in practice digoxin therapy is not a recognized contraindication to propranolol therapy *(Ch. 2, BNF)*.
d **True** Nocturnal dyspnoea indicates incipient heart failure. This is an important contraindication to propranolol therapy, which potentiates failure.
e **True** Postural hypotension may be associated with beta-blockade. A fully beta-blocked patient is unable to compensate with tachycardia in the presence of hypotension.

(Ch. 19, D)

a **True** This is a well-recognized side-effect, which can be prevented by administration of adequate doses of acetylcysteine.
b **False** Liver damage is not associated with acute overdose of aspirin.
c **False** Paraquat in acute overdosage causes a severe fibrotic reaction in the lungs but not liver damage *per se (Ch. Em, BNF)*.
d **False** Tricyclic antidepressant agents produce anticholinergic effects in overdosage; liver damage is not a feature *(Ch. Em, BNF)*.
e **False** In acute overdosage halothane causes cardiovascular and cerebral depression *(Ch. 8, A & S)*.

11 **A urine specific gravity of 1030 is compatible with**
 a diabetes insipidus.
 b diabetes mellitus.

 c normal renal function.
 d methoxyflurane nephrotoxicity.

 e syndrome of inappropriate antidiuretic hormone (ADH) secretion.

12 **Metabolic acidosis may be caused by**
 a implantation of the ureters into the colon.
 b hypoventilation.
 c acute renal failure.

 d pancreatic fistulae.

 e chronic diarrhoea.

13 **Aortic regurgitation is a common feature of**
 a Marfan's syndrome.

 b rheumatoid arthritis.

 c ankylosing spondylitis.

 d acromegaly.

 e thyrotoxicosis.

14 **In a patient with intestinal obstruction there may be**
 a an increased risk of pulmonary aspiration.

 b hyponatraemia.

 c hypovolaemia.

 d hyperkalaemia.

 e stimulation of ADH secretion if dehydration is present.

(Appendix VII, A & S)

a **False** A specific gravity of 1010 is expected in diabetes insipidus.
b **True** A specific gravity of 1030 is normal; in the absence of glycosuria, a patient with diabetes mellitus produces urine with normal specific gravity.
c **True** This value is within the normal range.
d **False** Methoxyflurane nephrotoxicity results in dilute urine and high-output renal failure.
e **False** Inappropriate secretion of ADH results in concentrated urine, with consequent water overload (Ch. 5, D).

(Ch. 21, A & S)

a **True** This may cause a hyperchloraemic acidosis.
b **False** This results in respiratory acidosis.
c **True** Metabolic acidosis is caused by inability to excrete hydrogen ions.
d **True** Loss of pancreatic juices results in loss of alkali and consequent metabolic acidosis.
e **True** Acidosis secondary to loss of bicarbonate may occur with chronic diarrhoea.

(Ch. 3, D)

a **True** Marfan's syndrome is a connective tissue disorder characterized by long thin extremities, high arched palate and subluxation of the lens. Dilatation of the first part of the aorta may occur, leading to aortic regurgitation.
b **False** Although rheumatoid granulomas may lead to aortic regurgitation, this is extremely rare (Ch. 12, D).
c **True** This is a well-recognized complication of ankylosing spondylitis (Ch. 12, D).
d **False** Cardiac failure occurs in acromegaly but this is not associated usually with aortic regurgitation.
e **False** A systolic aortic flow murmur may be present in thyrotoxicosis (Ch. 8, D).

(Ch. 31, A & S)

a **True** Vomiting, regurgitation and the possibility of aspiration always exist in a patient with intestinal obstruction.
b **True** Although hyponatraemia is possible, hypernatraemia or a normal serum sodium concentration are more usual in the presence of dehydration.
c **True** Loss of extracellular fluid into the bowel or by vomiting results in hypovolaemia.
d **False** If vomiting accompanies intestinal obstruction, loss of potassium and metabolic alkalosis may lead to hypokalaemia.
e **True** Secretion of ADH accompanies the stress response (Ch. 10, D).

15   In chronic obstructive airways disease (COAD)
a   the trachea descends on inspiration.

b   finger clubbing is a feature.

c   percussion of the heart border is an unreliable test of cardiomegaly.
d   the JVP may be raised.

e   the P wave of the ECG may be abnormal.

---

16   The following are true of anaphylaxis:
a   There is an increased incidence in atopic patients.

b   Hydrocortisone 200 mg is the first-line treatment.

c   Previous exposure to the offending agent is unusual.

d   Adrenaline should be administered.
e   It is less common following oral than following i.v. administration of the aetiological agent.

---

17   In sickle cell disease
a   individuals have either African or West Indian ancestry.

b   the Sickledex test is negative for the trait.

c   sickling occurs only at an oxygen tension < 2.9 kPa.

d   sickling is promoted by acidosis.

e   the crisis is precipitated by metabolic alkalosis.

---

18   In acute intermittent porphyria (AIP) the following drugs are contraindicated:
a   methohexitone.
b   sulphonamides.
c   chlorpropamide.

d   propofol.
e   NSAIDs.

(Ch. 4, D)

a **True** Tracheal descent on inspiration may be a feature of severe forms of emphysema.

b **False** Finger clubbing is a feature of suppurative lung disease and not COAD.

c **True** Because of the increased anteroposterior diameter of the chest and increased resting lung volume.

d **True** JVP may be raised if right heart failure complicates chronic obstructive airways disease.

e **True** An abnormal P wave (P pulmonale) occurs on the ECG because of enlargement of the right atrium.

(Ch. 22, A & S)

a **True** In atopic patients there is an increased serum concentration of IgE.

b **False** Hydrocortisone has no effect on immediate outcome and should be regarded as second-line therapy.

c **False** Previous exposure to the antigen is common in an anaphylactic reaction.

d **True** Adrenaline 50–100 μg should be administered.

e **True** With oral administration of an agent there is 'filtering' by the gastrointestinal tract.

(Ch. 11, D; Ch. 6, A & S)

a **False** The sickle cell gene is found also in those of Mediterranean origin or, less commonly, in those from the Indian subcontinent.

b **False** The Sickledex test is positive for both the trait (heterozygote) and the disease (homozygote).

c **False** Sickling in the homozygote occurs with oxygen tensions in the venous range (5–5.5 kPa).

d **True** Sickling is more likely to occur with low blood pH, high red cell 2,3-diphosphoglyceric acid (2,3-DPG) concentrations, stasis, dehydration and increased plasma osmolality.

e **False** Alkalosis is less likely to promote sickling of the abnormal red cells.

(Ch. 40, A & S)

a **True** All barbiturates are contraindicated in AIP.

b **True** The sulphonamides are contraindicated in AIP.

c **True** Chlorpropamide is a derivative of the sulphonamide group and is contraindicated in AIP.

d **False** Propofol does not precipitate an attack of AIP.

e **False** NSAIDs are regarded as safe in the presence of this disorder.

19 Reactions to blood transfusion usually include

a bronchospasm.

b laryngeal oedema.

c urticaria.

d facial oedema.

e myoglobinuria.

20 The following drugs are used currently to treat supraventricular tachycardia (SVT):

a verapamil.

b propranolol.

c lignocaine.

d nifedipine.

e neostigmine.

21 In acute severe hypovolaemia

a tidal volume increases.

b hyperventilation occurs.

c CO_2 retention occurs.

d ventilation/perfusion mismatch occurs.

e the oxyhaemoglobin dissociation curve shifts to the right.

(Ch. 11, D; Ch. 6, A & S)

a	**False**	Most transfusion reactions are haemolytic in nature. Anaphylactic reactions may occur; release of histamine would lead to marked bronchospasm, although this is rare.
b	**False**	This is a rare complication.
c	**True**	Urticarial weals or hives are thought to result from reaction between IgA and anti-IgA.
d	**False**	This is very rare.
e	**False**	Haemoglobinuria occurs commonly because of haemolysis, but myoglobinuria, caused by destruction of muscle myoglobin, does not occur.

(Ch. 13, A & S; Ch. 3, D)

a	**True**	Verapamil, a calcium-channel blocking drug, reduces the rate of spontaneous depolarization.
b	**True**	Beta-blockade facilitates unopposed vagal activity on the sinoatrial (SA) node.
c	**False**	Lignocaine is a membrane-stabilizing drug and has no effect on supraventricular arrhythmias.
d	**False**	Although nifedipine is a calcium-channel blocking drug, its predominant effects are peripheral and coronary vasodilatation.
e	**False**	Neostigmine has been superseded in this respect.

(Chs. 2 and 31, A & S)

a	**True**	Increased vasomotor centre activity radiates to the respiratory centre.
b	**True**	Increased peripheral chemoreceptor activity leads to stimulation of the respiratory centre.
c	**False**	There is hyperventilation and a decrease in Pa_{CO_2}.
d	**True**	Increased ventilation accompanied by a reduction in cardiac output and pulmonary artery pressure leads to an increase in $\dot{V}/\dot{Q}$ scatter. Oxygen therapy is important in the management of severe hypovolaemia.
e	**False**	Respiratory alkalosis shifts the oxyhaemoglobin dissociation curve to the left.

22 ABO blood group antigens
a   exhibit Mendelian inheritance.

b   are thought to be contained within red cells.

c   are absent in patients with blood group O.

d   are absent from leucocytes.
e   may be removed by washing red cells.

---

23 The following suggest acute massive pulmonary embolism:
a   accentuated mitral valve sounds.

b   elevated JVP.

c   deep Q waves and inverted T waves in lead I of the ECG.

d   cyanosis.

e   hepatojugular reflux.

---

24 Insulin requirements of diabetics increase
a   following onset of chronic renal failure.

b   during treatment with beta-blockers.

c   during the third trimester of pregnancy.

d   following the onset of diabetic gangrene.

e   during treatment with dopamine.

(Ch. 6, A & S)

a **True** The ABO blood groups described by Landsteiner exhibit Mendelian inheritance.

b **False** The antigenic elements of ABO blood groups are found on the surface of red cells.

c **True** The blood of group O patients contains antibodies to both A and B antigens.

d **True** The ABO system is a red cell system.

e **False** The washing of red cells is used to prevent HLA (human leukocyte antigen) incompatibility with white cells.

(Ch. 3, D)

a **False** In acute massive pulmonary embolism, there is wide splitting of the second heart sound, and a third sound may be heard over the right ventricle.

b **True** This invariably accompanies massive pulmonary embolism, because of right ventricular failure.

c **False** The ECG may show signs of acute right ventricular strain with an S wave in lead I and T wave inversion in V_1.

d **True** The combination of severe $\dot{V}/\dot{Q}$ mismatch and reduction in cardiac output results in cyanosis.

e **False** Hepatojugular reflux is a sign of long-standing right ventricular failure and liver congestion.

(Ch. 8, D)

a **False** Diabetic nephropathy may progress to chronic renal failure but diabetic management is unaffected.

b **True** Theoretically, beta-blockers may antagonize gluconeogenesis, but beta-blocker treatment may cause a reduction in glucose tolerance in diabetics and insulin requirements are increased (Ch. 40, A & S).

c **True** Insulin requirements increase during pregnancy. After parturition there may be a rapid decline.

d **True** The onset of infection produces insulin resistance and requirements increase.

e **True** This causes an increase in circulating catecholamine concentrations and impairment of glucose tolerance.

25 Rheumatoid arthritis
a may produce fixed flexion deformities of the neck.
b may be associated with mitral valve disease.
c may be associated with anaemia refractory to treatment.

d commonly involves the temporomandibular joint.

e is associated with discrete shadowing on the chest X-radiograph.

26 Gallstones are associated with the following:
a haemolytic anaemia.

b raised serum concentrations of bile salts.

c raised serum concentrations of calcium.

d hypoparathyroidism.

e pancreatic carcinoma.

27 Propranolol is contraindicated preoperatively if the following are present:
a left bundle branch block.

b orthopnoea or paroxysmal nocturnal dyspnoea.

c bronchial asthma.
d therapy with digoxin.
e therapy with verapamil.

28 Acute appendicitis may be mimicked by
a carcinoma of the caecum.

b herpes zoster.

c basal pneumonia.
d mesenteric adenitis.

e ectopic pregnancy.

(Ch. 40, A & S)

a	True	The cervical spine may be fixed or subluxed.
b	False	Rheumatoid arthritis is unrelated to rheumatic heart disease.
c	True	Chronic anaemia, either hypo- or normochromic, is common and this is refractory to iron therapy. In addition, NSAIDs may cause gastrointestinal haemorrhage.
d	True	The arthritic process may involve the temporomandibular joint, rendering laryngoscopy and intubation difficult.
e	True	There may be pulmonary involvement with interstitial fibrosis, producing $\dot{V}/\dot{Q}$ abnormalities and hypoxaemia.

(Ch. 10, D)

a	True	This results from increased quantities of products of haemoglobin metabolism.
b	True	25% of gallstones comprise pigment stones (calcium and bilirubinate).
c	False	Increased serum concentrations of calcium may cause renal stones.
d	False	Hypoparathyroidism leads to decreased serum concentrations of calcium; there is no association with gallstones.
e	False	There is no association between pancreatic carcinoma and gallstones.

(Ch. 12, A & S)

a	True	Left bundle branch block can progress to complete heart block in the presence of beta-blockade.
b	True	Propranolol is a myocardial depressant, and therefore contraindicated in the presence of left ventricular failure.
c	True	Propranolol is a non-cardioselective beta-blocker (Ch. 2, BNF).
d	False	But care should be exercised in the presence of cardiac failure.
e	True	The myocardial depressant actions of verapamil and beta-blockers are additive (Ch. 2, BNF).

(Ch. 9, D)

a	True	Acute appendicitis in adults may cause a mass in the right iliac fossa.
b	True	Prodromal symptoms of herpes zoster in the right T12/LI dermatomes may mimic the pain of acute appendicitis (Ch. 14, D).
c	True	Right basal pneumonia may produce pain in the right flank.
d	True	Non-specific mesenteric lymphadenitis may resemble appendicitis in children and adolescents.
e	True	But not in men!

29 Features of thyrotoxicosis in a young adult include
a low pulse pressure.
b large goitre.
c cold intolerance.
d menorrhagia.

e atrial fibrillation.

30 The causes of an increase in serum urea concentration after haematemesis include
a catabolism of blood in the gut.
b potassium loss.
c metabolic acidosis.
d hypovolaemia.

e dehydration.

31 Hypokalaemia
a causes enlarged P waves on the ECG.
b occurs in hyperaldosteronism.

c is a feature of Cushing's syndrome.
d is a feature of Cushing's disease.
e always reflects a decrease in total body potassium content.

32 Hyperkalaemia may be treated with
a intravenous insulin.

b intravenous calcium.

c oral ion-exchange resins.

d frusemide.

e glucocorticoids.

(Ch. 8, D)

a **False** Increased pulse pressure usually occurs.
b **False** There may be a goitre, but it is not usually large.
c **False** Cold intolerance is a feature of hypothyroidism.
d **True** Menorrhagia may be a presenting symptom in this condition; thyrotoxicosis is eight times more frequent in females than in males.
e **True** Thyrotoxicosis is a common non-cardiac cause of atrial fibrillation.

(Ch. 9, D)

a **True** Following red cell breakdown by intestinal bacteria.
b **False** Potassium loss does not influence serum urea concentration.
c **False** Serum urea concentration is not influenced by pH of blood.
d **True** Fluid loss from the extracellular space, but not hypovolaemia *per se*, causes an increase in serum urea concentration.
e **True** Dehydration from any cause may lead to increased serum urea concentration.

(Ch. 5, D; Ch. 21, A & S)

a **False** Hypokalaemia causes decreased T wave amplitude.
b **True** Excretion of K^+ is enhanced by aldosterone. Primary hyperaldosteronism is termed Conn's syndrome.
c **True** Excess mineralocorticoid activity promotes K^+ excretion.
d **True** See c above.
e **False** Hypokalaemia may be caused by compartmental shifts rather than loss from the body.

(Ch. 5, D; Ch. 21, A & S)

a **True** This enhances Na^+-K^+-ATPase activity and transfer of potassium from extra- to intracellular compartments.
b **True** This restores the Ca^{++}/K^+ ratio and stabilizes membranes, especially in cardiac muscle.
c **True** Calcium resonium 15 g, 6-hourly, is recommended, but is expensive and messy.
d **False** Although loop diuretics promote K^+ loss, this is not an initial treatment of choice. Hyperkalaemia may be the result of renal failure.
e **False** Glucocorticoids promote K^+ loss, but this action is not adequate for therapy.

33 Aortic stenosis may be caused by

a congenital anomalies.

b aortic valve calcification.
c ruptured aortic cusp.
d endocarditis.

e hypertrophic obstructive cardiomyopathy (HOCM).

34 The trachea may be deviated to the right in

a right upper lobe fibrosis.
b left simple pneumothorax.

c right pleural effusion.

d left lower lobar collapse.

e retrosternal goitre.

35 The risk of deep venous thrombosis (DVT) is increased by

a bedrest.
b anaemia.
c neoplastic disease.
d obesity.
e extradural anaesthesia.

36 Atrial fibrillation is associated with

a mitral stenosis.

b ischaemic heart disease.

c increased cardiac output.

d multiple P waves on the ECG.

e thrombus formation in the left atrial appendage.

(Ch. 3, D)

a **True** Aortic stenosis may result from premature calcification of a bicuspid aortic valve, or a subvalvular diaphragm.
b **True** This is common, especially in old age.
c **False** This results in aortic regurgitation.
d **False** This causes destruction of the valve leaflets, producing a systolic flow murmur and ultimately regurgitation.
e **False** The signs of HOCM are similar to those of aortic stenosis, but the obstruction is subvalvular.

(Ch. 4, D)

a **False** Fibrosis of the right upper lobe is unlikely to shift the trachea.
b **False** Deviation of the trachea to the right with a left pneumothorax occurs only if it is under tension.
c **False** Pleural effusions do not usually shift the trachea or mediastinum. If tracheal deviation is present, it would probably be to the left.
d **False** Left lower lobar collapse does not result in deviation of the trachea to the right.
e **True** The trachea may be deviated to left, right or not at all.

(Ch. 3, D)

a **True** Bedrest causes venous stasis (part of Virchow's triad).
b **False** Polycythaemia increases the risk of DVT.
c **True** Especially pelvic neoplasms.
d **True** This results from immobility.
e **False** Extradural anaesthesia has not been shown to increase risk of DVT, and may reduce it *(Ch. 25, A & S)*.

(Ch. 3, D)

a **True** Atrial dilatation, secondary to mitral stenosis, leads to atrial fibrillation.
b **True** Atrial fibrillation may be a sign of ischaemic heart disease in elderly patients.
c **False** Atrial contraction contributes approximately 20% to ventricular filling; cardiac output is reduced in atrial fibrillation.
d **False** Fibrillary waves characterize atrial fibrillation. P waves represent ordered depolarization.
e **True** Anticoagulant therapy may be advisable.

37 Hyperkalaemia is associated with
    a tall peaked T waves on the ECG.

    b U waves on the ECG.
    c enhanced digoxin toxicity.
    d pyloric stenosis.
    e haemolysis.

38 In chronic renal failure
    a the patient is symptomless until the glomerular filtration rate is less than 15 ml/min.
    b anaemia is common and must be corrected before surgery.

    c hypertension occurs because of secondary hyperaldosteronism.

    d suxamethonium is contraindicated because of hyperkalaemia.

    e enflurane is the volatile agent of choice during anaesthesia.

39 Serum concentrations of Na^+ 127 mmol/l, K^+ 6.0 mmol/l, urea 18 mmol/l, glucose 3 mmol/l, $NaHCO_3$ 18 mmol/l are compatible with
    a renal failure.

    b Addison's disease.

    c inappropriate secretion of ADH.

    d liver failure.

    e fluid overload.

40 In hepatocellular insufficiency the following occur:
    a hypokalaemia.
    b decreased plasma albumin concentration.
    c raised plasma bilirubin concentration.

    d decreased prothrombin time.

    e hyponatraemia.

(Ch. 21, A & S; Ch. 5, D)

a   **True**   Hyperkalaemia decreases the resting membrane potential.
Tall T waves are an early indication of an increased serum
potassium concentration.
b   **False**   U waves are associated with hypokalaemia.
c   **False**   Hyperkalaemia ameliorates digoxin toxicity.
d   **False**   Hypokalaemia may occur secondary to metabolic alkalosis.
e   **True**   Because of release of intracellular potassium.

(Ch. 6, D)

a   **True**   Slow deterioration of renal function may not be accompanied
by symptoms until a late stage in the disease.
b   **False**   Anaemia, though common, is well compensated and
preoperative transfusion should not be necessary. Prompt
treatment of intraoperative blood loss should take place.
c   **True**   Fluid retention also contributes. Patients often require
antihypertensive medication.
d   **True**   Further potassium release may occur, which is more hazardous
in the hyperkalaemic patient.
e   **False**   Enflurane is metabolized with the liberation of fluoride ions,
which may be nephrotoxic.

(Ch. 21, A & S; Ch. 5, D)

a   **True**   Hyperkalaemia, a low bicarbonate concentration, and a raised
urea concentration are typical of acute renal failure.
b   **True**   Addison's disease results in hyponatraemia, and renal failure
secondary to cardiac failure.
c   **False**   Water retention is the main feature of inappropriate ADH
secretion; serum sodium is usually lower and urea
concentration is reduced.
d   **False**   Liver failure is associated with hypokalaemia and diminished
production of urea.
e   **False**   A similar picture to that of inappropriate ADH secretion would
be seen.

(Ch. 10, D)

a   **True**   This is a result of impaired aldosterone metabolism.
b   **True**   Impaired synthesis of albumin is a feature of liver disease.
c   **True**   Conjugated and unconjugated bilirubin concentrations are
increased in hepatocellular jaundice.
d   **False**   The prothrombin time is increased because of impaired
synthesis of coagulation factors and decreased uptake of fat-
soluble vitamins.
e   **False**   Hypernatraemia occurs (see **a** above).

41 Hepatitis may be transmitted by

a cryoprecipitate.

b fibrinogen.

c fresh frozen plasma.

d anti-haemophilia globulin (factor VIII).

e purified beef gelatin.

42 Digoxin may be useful in

a atrial flutter.

b cardiac tamponade.

c paroxysmal supraventricular tachycardia.

d junctional rhythm.

e Prinzmetal's angina.

43 Acute renal failure

a is caused most commonly by acute ischaemia due to severe haemorrhage.

b may complicate the perioperative course of patients with jaundice.

c is associated with a urine:plasma urea ratio of 2:1 if the cause is prerenal.

d necessitates the insertion of a CVP catheter to monitor therapy.

e frequently results in persistent anuria.

44 Ventricular ectopic beats

a may cause heart failure.

b may convert to ventricular fibrillation in the presence of myocardial infarction.

c should always be treated.

d are indistinguishable from atrial extrasystoles at the radial pulse.

e may be treated with lignocaine.

(Ch. 6, A & S)

a	**True**	Cryoprecipitate may transmit hepatitis B virus *(Ch. 11, D)*.
b	**True**	Fibrinogen is obtained by cold precipitation of plasma with alcohol. Only products which have been heat-treated may be regarded as free from risk.
c	**True**	Fresh frozen plasma has not been heat-treated and contains many heat-labile coagulation factors.
d	**True**	Human AHG may transmit hepatitis, but genetically engineered AHG is now available.
e	**False**	The two gelatin solutions in common use (Gelofusine and Haemaccel) are free from hepatitis B virus.

(Ch. 3, D; Ch. 13, A & S)

a	**True**	Digoxin is used to control the ventricular rate in atrial flutter.
b	**False**	The treatment for cardiac tamponade is relief of the tamponade at the earliest opportunity.
c	**True**	Digoxin may be useful in paroxysmal supraventricular tachycardia, but beta-blocker or calcium-channel blocking drugs are now preferred.
d	**False**	Digoxin is contraindicated in junctional rhythm because it may increase block at the AV node.
e	**False**	The usual therapy for Prinzmetal's angina is administration of calcium-channel blocking drugs or beta-blockers.

(Ch. 6, D)

a	**True**	Oliguria occurs because of cortical vasoconstriction in response to diminished perfusion.
b	**True**	This is the hepatorenal syndrome.
c	**False**	The urine:plasma urea ratio frequently exceeds 10:1 in acute prerenal failure.
d	**True**	CVP should be monitored early, to permit control of intravascular resuscitation.
e	**False**	The urine output is sometimes normal, but tubular excretory function is impaired.

(Ch. 3, D)

a	**True**	There is a disturbance of stroke volume in addition to rhythm; this may cause heart failure.
b	**True**	After myocardial infarction, patients should be monitored and ventricular ectopic beats treated.
c	**False**	Ventricular ectopic beats may be benign, and occur in the normal individual.
d	**True**	The ECG is the only accurate means of diagnosing the origin of ectopic beats.
e	**True**	Lignocaine stabilizes membranes and suppresses ventricular ectopics.

45 With regard to actions of drugs on the heart

  a the effects of digoxin are potentiated by administration of calcium.

  b thiazide diuretics may precipitate digitalis toxicity.

  c digoxin is potentiated by hypoalbuminaemia.

  d digitoxin is the fastest-acting intravenous glycoside.

  e lignocaine is used usually for therapy of ventricular arrhythmias.

---

46 Hypokalaemia may occur in the presence of

  a metabolic acidosis.

  b respiratory acidosis.

  c rapid cellular uptake of glucose.

  d anuria.

  e extensive muscle breakdown.

---

47 Features of acute obstructive jaundice include

  a increased urinary urobilinogen concentration.

  b increased serum unconjugated bilirubin concentration.

  c increased faecal fat.

  d a palpable gall bladder, in which there would be stones.

  e alkaline phosphatase concentration exceeding 100 iu.

---

48 Features of acute small bowel obstruction include

  a nausea and vomiting.

  b central abdominal pain, worsened by movement.

  c abdominal distension.

  d dullness to percussion in the flanks.

  e low-pitched rumbling bowel sounds.

(Ch. 13, A & S; Ch. 3, D)

a **True** The action of digoxin is mediated by calcium.

b **True** Secondary to hypokalaemia induced by the diuretic.
c **True** This may result from diminished calcium-binding by albumin.
d **False** Digitoxin is not available for i.v. use.
e **True** Lignocaine is a Class I anti-arrhythmic drug.

(Ch. 21, A & S)

a **False** Acidosis causes a shift of potassium from the intracellular to the extracellular compartment.
b **False** See **a** above.
c **True** Secondary to insulin secretion, which drives extracellular potassium into the intracellular compartment.
d **False** Hyperkalaemia occurs in renal failure.
e **False** Intracellular potassium is released by damaged muscle.

(Ch. 10, D)

a **False** There is increased excretion of conjugated bilirubin.
b **False** But in long-standing cases, hepatocellular failure may occur.
c **True** Because of impaired excretion of bile salts, fat absorption is reduced.
d **False** Only severe obstruction caused by pancreatic carcinoma produces this sign.
e **True** This is diagnostic of biliary obstruction.

(Ch. 9, D; Ch. 31, A & S)

a **True** There is a risk of pulmonary aspiration preoperatively.
b **False** Pain of simple obstruction is usually colicky in nature.
c **False** Distension is associated with chronic large bowel obstruction.
d **False** This is a sign of ascites.
e **False** Characteristically, bowel sounds are increased and tinkling in nature.

49 An arterial plasma bicarbonate concentration of 18 mmol/l is consistent with

a   metabolic acidosis.

b   compensated metabolic acidosis.

c   compensated metabolic alkalosis.

d   compensated respiratory alkalosis.

e   respiratory acidosis.

50 The following feature is characteristic of the accompanying cardiac abnormality:

a   tapping apex beat in mitral incompetence.

b   right atrial hypertrophy in mitral stenosis.

c   collapsing pulse in aortic stenosis.
d   diastolic murmur at the left sternal edge in aortic incompetence.
e   cyanosis in congenital heart disease with right-to-left shunt.

51 Diagnosis of brain stem death in the UK requires

a   absence of spinal reflexes.

b   flat EEG.
c   no ventilatory movement when Pa_{CO_2} exceeds 7 kPa.
d   no gag reflex following passage of a suction catheter down the trachea.
e   absence of contrast medium in anterior and middle cerebral arteries on carotid angiography.

52 In tetanus

a   reflex hyperactivity occurs.

b   ST and T wave changes occur on the ECG because of toxic myocarditis.
c   the relaxant of choice for IPPV (intermittent positive-pressure ventilation) is pancuronium.
d   prognosis is independent of incubation period.
e   tracheostomy is always indicated.

(Ch. 5, D; Ch. 21, A & S)

a	**True**	An excess of hydrogen ions drives the carbonic acid/bicarbonate equilibrium to the left.
b	**True**	A reduction in bicarbonate ion concentration defines metabolic acidosis.
c	**False**	A plasma bicarbonate concentration of 18 mmol/l indicates moderate to severe metabolic acidosis.
d	**True**	Renal compensatory mechanisms excrete sodium and bicarbonate ions in respiratory alkalosis.
e	**False**	Hydrogen ion concentration and Pa_{CO_2} are increased, and HCO_3^- is normal or slightly elevated.

(Ch. 3, D)

a	**False**	Rapid closure of the mitral valve in mitral stenosis may produce a tapping quality.
b	**True**	This may be manifest as a prominent 'a' wave in the jugular venous pulse.
c	**False**	This is characteristic of aortic incompetence.
d	**True**	Heard best during expiration with the patient leaning forward.
e	**True**	Desaturated blood reaches the systemic circulation.

(Ch. 41, A & S)

a	**False**	Spinal reflexes may occur in the absence of brain stem integrity.
b	**False**	The EEG is not required as part of the protocol in the UK.
c	**True**	The Pa_{CO_2}, must be checked.
d	**True**	There should be no response to passage of a suction catheter into the nose, mouth or bronchial tree.
e	**False**	Angiography is unnecessary.

(Ch. 14, D)

a	**True**	The exotoxin has an affinity for motor nerve endings and anterior horn cells.
b	**False**	But autonomic nerve involvement may cause cardiovascular complications.
c	**False**	Hypertension may complicate the disease and this would be worsened by pancuronium.
d	**False**	The shorter the incubation period, the more severe the attacks.
e	**False**	Local tetanus may affect only the muscles near the infected wound.

53 Myasthenia gravis

a is probably an autoimmune disease.

b exhibits increased sensitivity to non-depolarizing and depolarizing relaxants.

c resembles myasthenic syndrome in the response to muscle relaxants.

d requires thymectomy only in patients exceeding 50 years of age with a thymoma.

e is exacerbated by ACTH therapy before there is improvement.

54 Extradural haemorrhage

a often results from a tear in the middle meningeal artery.

b if severe enough to cause clinical signs, causes hemiplegia on the same side as the haemorrhage.

c initially causes pupillary dilation, on the same side as the haemorrhage.

d is often followed by a lucid interval after a period of concussion.

e is often bilateral, in common with subdural haematomas.

55 Inhalation of large food particles rapidly causes

a cyanosis.

b asphyxia.

c mediastinal shift.

d pneumothorax.

e bronchospasm.

56 Concerning hip fractures in the elderly

a pulmonary embolus is the most common cause of death.

b a delay of 7–10 days before surgery is beneficial.

c spinal anaesthesia is a useful alternative to general anaesthesia.

d spinal anaesthesia decreases mortality in comparison with general anaesthesia.

e all patients are hypoxic in the immediate postoperative period, irrespective of anaesthetic technique.

(Ch. 40, A & S; Ch. 14, D)

a	**True**	The number of acetylcholine receptors is diminished because of an autoimmune reaction between the receptor and an antibody.
b	**False**	The response to depolarizing relaxants may be variable, but is often normal.
c	**False**	There is sensitivity to all relaxants in myasthenic syndrome.
d	**False**	Thymectomy is effective in the early stages of the disease.
e	**True**	Steroid treatment is not recommended as the initial treatment.

(Ch. 14, D)

a	**True**	The artery is superficial and susceptible to injury.
b	**False**	Usually contralateral hemiplegia occurs.
c	**False**	Ipsilateral pupillary dilation is a late sign, produced by third nerve compression.
d	**True**	There is a danger in discharging a patient during this time.
e	**False**	Unilateral injury is more common.

(Ch. 31, A & S)

a	**True**	Large food particles may cause upper airway obstruction and asphyxia.
b	**True**	See **a** above.
c	**False**	Mediastinal movement is not an early feature in the acute phase of inhalation of large particles.
d	**False**	Pneumothorax is unlikely in this situation.
e	**True**	Unsuspected aspiration of stomach contents on induction of anaesthesia or during the course of anaesthesia may precipitate bronchospasm.

(Chs. 23 and 26, A & S)

a	**False**	Bronchopneumonia is the most common cause of death in these patients.
b	**False**	Although some immediate resuscitation may be required, in general the earlier the operation is performed, the better the outlook.
c	**True**	However, care has to be taken to avoid the hypotension which may accompany spinal anaesthesia in an emergency anaesthetic.
d	**False**	Although there is a significant difference in mortality in the first 4 weeks after surgery, there is no long-term difference following spinal or general anaesthesia.
e	**False**	Hypoxaemia occurs immediately after anaesthesia following the use of nitrous oxide, but not after spinal anaesthesia.

57   In chronic bronchitis
a   there is usually a history of chronic smoke inhalation.

b   mucus secretion is increased.

c   the ratio FEV_1/FVC is normal.
d   the 10-year survival rate is poor.

e   residual volume (RV) is reduced.

---

58   The following are associated with a low fixed cardiac output:
a   aortic regurgitation.

b   aortic stenosis.
c   mitral stenosis.

d   mild hypothyroidism.

e   digoxin toxicity.

---

59   A patient with a long-standing paralysis caused by transection of the spinal cord at T5
a   has flaccid legs.

b   is poikilothermic.
c   has a mass autonomic reflex.

d   has a reduction in FVC.

e   may demonstrate a large increase in serum K^+ concentration in response to suxamethonium.

---

60   The following are features of cervical sympathetic chain damage:
a   enophthalmos.
b   miosis.
c   dilated conjunctival vessels.
d   congested nasal mucosa.

e   ptosis.

(Ch. 4, D)

a **True** Chronic bronchitis is much more common in smokers than in non-smokers.

b **True** There is overactivity of the mucus-secreting glands in the bronchi and bronchioles.

c **False** FEV_1 is reduced and the ratio of FEV_1 to FVC is also reduced.

d **False** Patients may survive for many years, though with gradually diminishing respiratory reserve.

e **False** Residual volume may be increased because of air trapping.

(Ch. 3, D)

a **False** The left ventricular stroke volume may be two to three times normal, but aortic flow may be reduced because of valvular regurgitation.

b **True** Restricted cardiac output may result in syncope on exercise.

c **True** The reduced left ventricular output may result in pulmonary oedema.

d **False** Basal metabolic rate is reduced but the cardiac output, although reduced, is not necessarily fixed. Cardiac failure may occur in the later stages *(Ch. 8, D)*.

e **False** Bradycardia and coupled ventricular extrasystoles may occur.

(Ch. 14, D)

a **False** With transection of the spinal cord at T5, there would be spastic paralysis.

b **False** The thermoregulatory centre is not affected.

c **True** The mass reflex comprises urination, defaecation, sweating and cardiovascular lability; it occurs in patients with chronic paraplegia.

d **True** Loss of the use of the lower thoracic muscles in expiration results in a decrease in FVC.

e **False** The rise in potassium associated with suxamethonium is a transient phenomenon which occurs between approximately 24 h and 6 months after denervation injuries *(Ch. 40, A & S)*.

(Ch. 14, D)

a **True** This is a feature of Horner's syndrome.

b **True** This is a feature of Horner's syndrome.

c **True** This results from lack of sympathetically induced vasoconstriction.

d **True** The sympathetic supply to the nose causes vasoconstriction – thus sympathetic block or damage causes vasodilatation.

e **True** The levator palpebrae superioris is innervated partly by the sympathetic system, and ptosis may therefore result from damage to the sympathetic supply.

61 Hypothyroidism

a is accompanied rarely by symptoms of myxoedema.

b is complicated by ulnar nerve compression and tingling in the fingers.

c may result in difficulty with tracheal intubation because of tongue enlargement.

d is occasionally accompanied by a pericardial effusion, which is visible on X-ray.

e results in a decrease in cardiac output.

---

62 A patient with a serum Na^+ concentration of 125 mmol/l and K^+ concentration of 6.1 mmol/l has features compatible with

a hypopituitarism.

b Addison's disease.

c hyperaldosteronism.

d Cushing's syndrome.

e inappropriate secretion of ADH.

---

63 In a comatose diabetic patient, the following are more likely to be features of hypoglycaemia than of ketoacidosis:

a dry mucous membranes.

b extensor plantar response.

c hyperventilation.

d hypotension.

e sweating.

---

64 Warming stored blood immediately before transfusion

a is associated with an increased incidence of infection.

b increases CO_2 content.

c increases O_2 content.

d is associated with a lower incidence of arrhythmias.

e shifts the oxyhaemoglobin dissociation curve to the right.

(Ch. 8, D)

a	**False**	Myxoedema often, but not invariably, accompanies hypothyroidism.
b	**False**	Carpal tunnel compression of the median nerve is associated with hypothyroidism.
c	**True**	Tongue enlargement is a feature of hypothyroidism and may render laryngoscopy difficult.
d	**True**	Cardiomegaly and a pericardial effusion may be present. The effusion usually resolves with treatment of the hypothyroidism.
e	**True**	Cardiac output and basal metabolic rate are reduced. Drug distribution and metabolism are affected.

(Ch. 8, D)

a	**True**	Hypopituitarism leads to an Addisonian crisis because of absence of secretion of ACTH.
b	**True**	These results are characteristic of an Addisonian patient.
c	**False**	Hyperaldosteronism causes hypernatraemia and hypokalaemia – Conn's syndrome.
d	**False**	In Cushing's syndrome, there is sodium retention and loss of potassium.
e	**False**	Although increased ADH secretion results in hyponatraemia, hyperkalaemia is not a feature.

(Ch. 8, D)

a	**False**	Ketoacidosis is accompanied by dehydration, which causes dry mucous membranes.
b	**True**	Brisk extensor plantar reflexes accompany hypoglycaemic coma.
c	**False**	Hyperventilation (Kussmaul's respiration) is one of the characteristic features of ketoacidosis.
d	**False**	Hypotension occurs in ketoacidosis because of loss of extracellular fluid.
e	**True**	Hypoglycaemia is associated with increased sympatho-adrenal activity.

(Ch. 31, A & S)

a	**False**	There is no increased incidence of infection associated with the use of blood warmers.
b	**False**	Carriage of CO_2 is uninfluenced.
c	**False**	The solubility of oxygen in plasma decreases with increased temperature. Oxygen carriage in whole blood is unchanged.
d	**True**	Transfusion of cold blood may produce arrhythmias. Warming blood before transfusion obviates this risk.
e	**True**	The oxyhaemoglobin dissociation curve is shifted to the right by increasing temperature.

65 Systemic arterial pressure may be overestimated by sphygmomanometry if

a   the cuff is too small for the arm.

b   the patient has severe arteriosclerosis.

c   the cuff is deflated very slowly.

d   the sphygmomanometer is at a higher level than the patient.

e   the patient is obese.

---

66 In a state of water intoxication, the following are true:

a   A low serum sodium concentration is present.

b   There may be a low urine output.

c   There is increased right atrial pressure.

d   Increased body weight is present.

e   Treatment with frusemide 80 mg is indicated.

---

67 In a patient with jaundice, a serum alkaline phosphatase concentration of 300 iu/l suggests

a   the presence of a hepatoma.

b   hepatocellular dysfunction.

c   biliary obstruction.
d   cholangitis.
e   that gamma-glutamyl transferase (γ-GT) concentration is always elevated.

(Ch. 20, A & S)

a **True** If the cuff is too narrow the arterial pressure may be overestimated. The cuff should cover two-thirds of the length of the upper arm.
b **True** In this case, the pulse pressure also tends to be abnormally high *(Ch. 3, D)*.
c **False** The converse is true. Rapid deflation tends to result in overestimation.
d **False** The column of air in the tube between the patient and the mercury manometer has little influence.
e **True** A larger cuff than usual may be required in an obese patient.

(Ch. 21, A & S; Ch. 5, D)

a **True** Water intoxication dilutes plasma sodium concentration and reduces plasma osmolality.
b **True** This may result from inappropriate secretion of ADH or renal damage.
c **True** Water retention causes increased extracellular fluid (ECF) (and plasma) volume. Stimulation of right atrial receptors suppresses ADH secretion and causes diuresis.
d **True** Weight is used frequently to monitor haemodialysis in patients with renal failure.
e **False** Therapy consists of treatment of the underlying cause, restricting water intake and, in severe cases, administration of 5% sodium chloride.

(Ch. 10, D)

a **False** Alpha-fetoprotein concentration is elevated in association with hepatoma.
b **False** Alkaline phosphatase concentration increases with biliary obstruction.
c **True** See **b** above.
d **True** A picture of biliary obstruction is produced.
e **True** Elevation of gamma-glutamyl transferase concentration occurs in biliary obstruction. It is a sensitive index of liver abnormality.

68 Raynaud's disease

a responds consistently to vasodilators.

b affects fingers more often than toes.

c never causes irreversible ischaemia.

d presents with pain as the commonest symptom.

e may be associated with cryoglobulinaemia.

69 Peripheral deep vein thrombosis

a is associated commonly with chronic non-malignant medical conditions.

b is associated with malignancy.

c comprises platelet thrombus.

d may lead to acute cor pulmonale.

e is associated with thrombocytopenia.

70 In fat embolism the following features may be present:

a pyrexia.

b fat globules in the sputum.
c fat globules in the urine.
d petechiae.
e reduced Pa_{O_2}.

71 Pleural effusion is a common complication of

a staphylococcal pneumonia.

b streptococcal pneumonia.

c *Mycoplasma* pneumonia.

d viral pneumonia.

e pneumococcal pneumonia.

(Ch. 3, D)

a **False** Although nifedipine may be useful, the response to vasodilators is not universally successful.

b **True** The disorder is usually bilateral, and fingers are affected more than toes.

c **False** In the later stages, ischaemic changes of the digits and gangrene may occur.

d **False** Numbness, tingling and burning are more common presenting features than pain.

e **True** Cryoglobulins occur in association with secondary Raynaud's disease or phenomenon.

(Ch. 3, D)

a **False** Peripheral thrombosis is not a common feature of chronic medical disease *per se*.

b **True** Increased blood coagulability may occur in malignant disease.

c **False** Although platelet thrombus may initiate the process, fibrin and red cells are the elements of the thrombus.

d **True** Pulmonary thromboembolism may produce acute right heart failure.

e **False** Increases in platelets and platelet adhesiveness are factors which promote venous thrombosis.

(Ch. 41, A & S)

a **True** Dyspnoea, cyanosis and pyrexia may occur as a result of pulmonary fat embolism.

b **True**

c **True**

d **True** Particularly in the upper chest, neck and conjunctivae.

e **True** Because of increased $\dot{V}/\dot{Q}$ scatter, Pa_{O_2} may be low even in the presence of a high inspired oxygen concentration.

(Ch. 4, D)

a **False** Staphylococcal pneumonia may occur as a complication of influenza or as suppurative pneumonia. Pleural reaction and effusion are not common in these conditions.

b **True** Streptococcal pneumonia is the most common type of primary pneumonia; pleural effusion may complicate this.

c **False** The pneumonia of *Mycoplasma* produces fewer clinical signs than classical pneumonia.

d **False** The physical signs of viral pneumonia are less marked than those of bacterial pneumonia, and pleural effusion is not common.

e **True** Pleural effusion may complicate classical pneumococcal pneumonia.

72 **Jaundice without bilirubinuria may result from**
   a Gilbert's syndrome.
   b infective hepatitis.

   c bile duct obstruction.
   d haemolytic anaemia.

   e metastatic liver secondaries.

---

73 **The insulin-dependent diabetic perioperatively**
   a must receive short-acting insulin therapy on the day before surgery to achieve stabilization.

   b may exhibit proteinuria as a result of diabetic nephropathy.

   c should have preoperative measurements of arterial blood pressure in the supine and erect positions.

   d requires less insulin if blood transfusion is required.

   e may receive low-dose insulin infusion without concurrent glucose administration.

---

74 **An i.v. infusion of dopamine 10 μg/kg per min produces an increase in**
   a cardiac output.

   b renal blood flow.

   c systemic vascular resistance.

   d urine output.

   e urinary sodium excretion.

(Ch. 10, D)

a **True**

b **True** Hepatocellular damage results in loss of conjugation of bilirubin. Only conjugated bilirubin is found in the urine, because it is water-soluble.

c **False** Conjugated bilirubin is available for urinary excretion.

d **True** Unconjugated bilirubin is the cause of jaundice in haemolytic anaemia.

e **False** There is a large reserve of liver function, and conjugation is maintained until a very late stage of metastatic spread.

(Ch. 40, A & S; Ch. 8, D)

a **False** Well-controlled diabetics on moderate doses of long-acting insulin may be managed safely on the day before surgery without changing the regimen.

b **True** Proteinuria signifies increasing renal failure. Accompanying hypertension should be controlled.

c **True** Variation between supine and erect arterial pressure may indicate the presence of autonomic neuropathy. Severe hypotension may complicate IPPV (intermittent positive-pressure ventilation).

d **False** Blood transfusion and Hartmann's solution increase insulin requirements because lactate stimulates gluconeogenesis.

e **True** Whilst this may be adequate for minor surgery of short duration, insulin and glucose combinations are usually prescribed.

(Ch. 12, Appx III b, A & S)

a **True** Dopamine in this dosage has a positive inotropic effect but causes little or no peripheral vasoconstriction.

b **True** Reduction in renal arterial resistance results in increased renal blood flow and glomerular filtration rate.

c **False** There is little or no peripheral vasoconstrictor effect in this dosage.

d **True** An increase in urine output occurs as a result of the renal and inotropic effects of dopamine.

e **True** Increases in renal blood flow, glomerular filtration rate and sodium excretion occur with low and medium doses of dopamine.

75 **Fluid overload may cause**

   a an increase in urine output.
   b an increase in CVP.
   c increased lung compliance.

   d dependent oedema.
   e hepatojugular reflux.

76 **In a young female patient with a history of asthma, presenting for minor surgery under general anaesthesia**

   a a history of atopy and allergy is likely.

   b high-pitched inspiratory rhonchi would be heard on auscultation of the chest.
   c perioperative steroid cover should be given if the patient has received steroids in the previous 6 months.

   d halothane is the preferred volatile agent.
   e high concentrations of oxygen are safe if administered postoperatively.

77 **The following drugs instilled into the conjunctival sac cause mydriasis:**

   a ephedrine.

   b timolol.

   c amethocaine.
   d homatropine.
   e cocaine.

78 **Chronic adrenal insufficiency leads to**

   a hyponatraemia.
   b hypokalaemia.
   c hypovolaemia.
   d hypotension.

   e hypoglycaemia.

(Chs. 3 and 21, A & S)

a **True** This is the normal physiological method of fluid regulation.
b **True** Fluid overload leads to an increase in CVP.
c **False** A decrease in lung compliance occurs with pulmonary oedema secondary to fluid overload.
d **True** Dependent oedema is a sign of fluid overload.
e **True** When venous pressure is increased transiently by pressure on the abdomen, the level of pulsation moves upwards in the neck – hepatojugular reflux *(Ch. 3, D)*.

(Ch. 40, A & S; Ch. 4, D)

a **True** 'Early onset' asthma occurs more commonly in atopic individuals.
b **False** Prolonged expiration and expiratory rhonchi are the hallmarks of asthma.
c **False** For minor surgery in the case of a patient not taking steroids, this is unnecessary. However, close postoperative supervision is essential and steroid treatment should be considered if symptoms dictate.
d **True** Halothane possesses bronchodilator properties.
e **True** There is no loss of central CO_2 response in patients with asthma alone.

(Ch. 11, BNF)

a **True** This is caused by stimulation of the beta-adrenoceptors in the dilator pupillae.
b **False** Timolol causes pupillary constriction and is used in the treatment of glaucoma.
c **False** Amethocaine is a local anaesthetic.
d **True** Homatropine is a shorter-acting mydriatic agent than atropine.
e **True** Cocaine has sympathomimetic actions.

(Ch. 8, D)

a **True** Because of absence of mineralocorticoid activity.
b **False** Hyperkalaemia occurs in Addison's disease.
c **True** This occurs because of excessive sodium and water losses.
d **True** Hypotension accompanies hypovolaemia. Normal reflex maintenance of arterial pressure is impaired also, and postural hypotension may be particularly troublesome.
e **True** Reactive hypoglycaemia may occur after a carbohydrate meal. Cortisol is one of the physiological antagonists of insulin.

79 **The following may be features of acute myocardial infarction:**
a basal crepitations.

b epigastric pain.

c absence of pain.
d effective pain relief with glyceryl trinitrate (GTN).
e dyspnoea.

80 **Abnormal patterns may occur in lead V_5 of the ECG in**
a anterior mural ischaemia.
b lateral wall ischaemia.
c inferior ventricular ischaemia.
d posterior ventricular ischaemia.
e transmural infarct.

81 **After cardiac arrest following acute myocardial infarction (MI):**
a lignocaine is indicated for prevention of atrial tachycardia.

b oxygen should be given by mask or nasal prongs.

c defibrillation is likely to be effective.

d $NaHCO_3$ 200 mmol is indicated.

e $NaHCO_3$ 1 mmol/kg is recommended.

82 **The following arrhythmias in an adult are treated in the acute situation by the accompanying therapy:**
a sinus bradycardia – atropine 0.6 mg i.v.
b ventricular tachycardia – lignocaine 100 mg i.v.

c asystole – adrenaline 0.05 mg i.v.
d atrial flutter – cardioversion.

e sinus tachycardia – verapamil 5 mg i.v.

(Ch. 3, D)

a	**True**	Basal crepitations signify left ventricular failure, which may complicate acute myocardial infarction.
b	**True**	The pain of acute myocardial infarction may be perceived in the epigastrium.
c	**True**	Myocardial infarction may be painless.
d	**False**	GTN does not relieve the pain of acute myocardial infarction.
e	**True**	'Cardiac asthma' (acute left ventricular failure) may be associated with acute myocardial infarction.

(Ch. 3, D)

a	**False**	Changes occur in leads V_2–V_4.
b	**True**	Left-sided chest leads reflect lateral ischaemic changes.
c	**False**	Leads II, III and aVF usually show inferior ischaemia.
d	**False**	Changes would be seen only in leads V_1 and V_4.
e	**True**	Q waves would be present in a lateral transmural infarction.

(Ch. 43, A & S; Ch. 3, D)

a	**False**	Lignocaine may be indicated to prevent recurrence of ventricular fibrillation.
b	**True**	Gas transfer may be impaired and the patient may be hypotensive.
c	**True**	Cardiac arrest after acute MI is likely to be caused by ventricular fibrillation. This is more common than asystole.
d	**False**	In the absence of metabolic acidosis, bicarbonate is not indicated.
e	**False**	Bicarbonate adds a significant sodium load and increases Pa_{CO_2}.

(Chs. 13 and 43, A & S)

a	**True**	Atropine is an antimuscarinic.
b	**True**	The membrane-stabilizing action of lignocaine is appropriate for ventricular arrhythmias.
c	**False**	1 mg (1000 μg) is appropriate.
d	**True**	Cardioversion is the most appropriate initial treatment. Digoxin is second-line therapy.
e	**False**	Verapamil is not the agent of first choice for sinus tachycardia. A beta-blocker such as metoprolol might be appropriate treatment if carotid sinus massage fails.

83 **The following are not associated with increased water loss:**
a diabetes insipidus.
b acute tubular necrosis.
c strenuous exercise.

d inappropriate secretion of ADH.
e treatment with carbonic anhydrase inhibitors.

---

84 **The following are indicated in the management of a patient who has taken an overdose of tricyclic antidepressants:**
a immediate i.v. administration of a beta-blocker.

b measurement of serum tricyclic concentration.

c forced acid diuresis.
d diazepam.

e pyridostigmine.

---

85 **With respect to carbon monoxide poisoning**
a infants are at greater risk than adults.
b toxicity occurs at carboxyhaemoglobin concentrations of less than 5%.
c cardiorespiratory arrest may occur.
d toxicity never occurs with inhalation of natural gas.

e hyperbaric oxygen treatment is useful.

---

86 **In paracetamol overdose**
a coma is uncommon.
b hypoglycaemia is a danger.
c prothrombin time may increase.

d haemofiltration is a useful measure.

e acetylcysteine therapy is indicated.

(Ch. 5, D)

a	**False**	Diabetes is associated classically with water loss.
b	**True**	Oliguria is a normal feature of acute tubular necrosis.
c	**False**	During severe exercise, sweating may deplete total body water by several litres.
d	**True**	ADH produces water retention.
e	**False**	Carbonic anhydrase inhibitors act as diuretic agents.

(Ch. 19, D; Ch. Em, BNF)

a	**False**	Tachyarrhythmias associated with tricyclic antidepressant overdose are treated most appropriately with physostigmine.
b	**False**	There is no indication for measuring tricyclic antidepressant concentrations in the treatment of poisoning.
c	**False**	Forced acid diuresis is an inappropriate therapy.
d	**True**	Diazepam may be used to reduce cerebral irritability, which is a feature in some patients.
e	**False**	Pyridostigmine has weak antimuscarinic effects and does not cross the blood–brain barrier.

(Ch. 19, D)

a	**True**	
b	**False**	Carboxyhaemoglobin concentrations of up to 5% have been recorded in cigarette smokers.
c	**True**	Failure of oxygen delivery to the tissues results in hypoxaemia.
d	**True**	There is no carbon monoxide in natural gas. However, carbon monoxide may be released if there is incomplete combustion of natural gas.
e	**True**	Hyperbaric oxygen increases the rate of elimination of carbon monoxide.

(Ch. 19, D; Ch. Em, BNF)

a	**True**	Coma is not a common feature of paracetamol overdose.
b	**True**	This may occur after an interval of approximately 36 h.
c	**True**	Because of inhibition of synthesis secondary to hepatic damage.
d	**False**	Haemofiltration is not indicated. However, haemoperfusion and/or haemodialysis may be indicated in the presence of liver or renal failure.
e	**True**	Acetylcysteine and methionine may protect the liver if given within 10–12 h of ingestion of paracetamol.

87 **A pulmonary artery catheter may be used**
a to assess left atrial pressure.

b to diagnose pulmonary hypertension.

c to measure left ventricular output.

d only via the internal jugular vein.

e with a dye dilution technique to measure cardiac output.

88 **In carcinoma of the head of the pancreas**
a painless jaundice is a common feature.
b preoperative glucose tolerance testing is indicated.

c serum acid phosphatase concentration is increased.

d perioperative treatment with mannitol is indicated.

e the 1-year survival is less than 10%.

89 **Dextran**
a affects coagulation.

b is allergenic.

c causes rouleaux formation if mixed with blood.

d may cause renal damage.
e may interfere with crossmatching.

90 **CPD (citrate phosphate dextrose) blood which has been stored for 21 days**
a is rich in platelets.
b has a normal 2,3-DPG concentration.

c has a high lactate concentration.

d has a high extracellular K^+ concentration.

e contains extracellular haemoglobin.

(Ch. 20, A & S)

a **True** Pulmonary capillary wedge pressure is related to left atrial pressure, and may be measured with this device.
b **True** Pulmonary arterial pressure may be measured (normally 25/10 mmHg).
c **True** A thermodilution catheter may be used to measure the output of the right ventricle, which is equal (within 1%) to the left ventricular output.
d **False** Any large vein will suffice, although the internal jugular vein is convenient.
e **False** Thermodilution is the technique usually employed. A pulmonary artery catheter cannot be used alone to measure cardiac output by dye dilution; peripheral blood sampling is required also.

(Ch. 9, D)

a **True**
b **True** An abnormal glucose tolerance test may be encountered preoperatively in a patient in whom this diagnosis is suspected.
c **False** Serum alkaline phosphatase is increased in carcinoma of the head of the pancreas.
d **True** Perioperative administration of mannitol is thought to decrease the likelihood of the hepatorenal syndrome developing.
e **True** The prognosis is very poor.

(Ch. 6, A & S)

a **True** Dextran has been used for its anticoagulant properties in the prevention of DVT.
b **True** The incidence of hypersensitivity reactions to i.v. administration of dextran is approximately 0.3%.
c **True** Formation of rouleaux after mixing with blood interferes with cross-matching.
d **True** Dextran 40 has been implicated in renal damage.
e **True** See **c** above.

(Chs. 6 and 31, A & S)

a **False** Platelet numbers and function deteriorate after 24 h of storage.
b **False** There is 20% loss of 2,3-DPG after 2 weeks' storage. Levels are not restored to normal until 24 h after transfusion.
c **True** The presence of high concentrations of lactic acid contributes to the low pH of stored blood.
d **True** Extracellular potassium concentration may be considerably higher than that of normal blood – up to 25 mmol/l.
e **True** Haemolysis in vitro results in an increase in extracellular haemoglobin concentration.

91 **In chronic obstructive airways disease, a 'pink puffer' differs from a 'blue bloater' in having a lower**

   a FEV_1.

   b number of red blood cells.

   c base excess.

   d FRC.

   e Pa_{O_2}.

92 **An increased serum concentration of alkaline phosphatase is found in the following:**

   a obstructive jaundice.

   b Paget's disease.
   c osteoporosis.
   d haemolytic anaemia.

   e prostatic carcinoma.

93 **Peripheral nerve injury is likely to occur in**
   a mid-forearm fracture involving both bones.

   b a midshaft fracture of the humerus.
   c dislocated shoulder.

   d the lithotomy position.

   e midshaft fracture of the femur.

94 **In chronic anaemia (Hb < 5 g/dl), the patient compensates with**
   a increased cardiac output.
   b decreased blood volume.

   c hyperventilation at rest.

   d shift of the oxyhaemoglobin dissociation curve (ODC) to the left.
   e decrease in red cell 2,3-DPG concentration.

(Ch. 4, D; Ch. 40, A & S)

a **False** In both groups of patients with chronic obstructive airways disease, the FEV_1 is reduced.
b **True** In chronic hypoxaemia and type II respiratory failure, polycythaemia may supervene.
c **True** Hypercapnia produces a compensatory non-respiratory alkalosis.
d **False** In emphysema, destruction of lung tissue and increase in the anteroposterior diameter of the chest increase FRC.
e **False** Hypoxaemia characterizes the bronchitic 'blue bloater'.

(Ch. 10, D)

a **True** Increased serum alkaline phosphatase concentration is a feature of obstructive jaundice.
b **True** This is caused by osteoblastic activity *(Ch. 12, D)*.
c **False** Osteoblastic activity is not a feature of osteoporosis.
d **False** Haemolytic activity itself does not result in alterations in serum alkaline phosphatase concentration.
e **False** This is associated classically with an increased acid phosphatase concentration, but secondary prostatic carcinoma may be associated with increased alkaline phosphatase concentration.

---

a **False** The median and ulnar nerves are more vulnerable in wrist and elbow injuries.
b **True** The radial nerve may be involved in a midshaft humeral fracture.
c **True** The cords of the brachial plexus lie in close proximity and may be involved in shoulder dislocations *(Ch. 25, A & S)*.
d **True** A misplaced leg support may result in compression of the lateral popliteal nerve *(Ch. 19, A & S)*.
e **False** The femoral nerve branches proximal to the midshaft of the femur. The sciatic nerve is well-protected by muscles.

(Ch. 6, A & S; Ch. 11, D)

a **True** Both stroke volume and heart rate increase.
b **False** With a chronic reduction in red cell mass, there is an accompanying increase in plasma volume; blood volume is unchanged.
c **False** The clinical features of chronic anaemia reflect the diminished oxygen-carrying capacity of the blood. Hyperventilation is not present at rest, but there is dyspnoea on exertion *(Ch. 11, D)*.
d **False** The ODC is shifted to the right in chronic anaemia (see **e** below).
e **False** There is increased synthesis of 2,3-DPG, which is responsible for the shift of the ODC to the right.

95 **A low serum sodium concentration accompanied by low total body sodium content occurs in**

a heart failure with oedema.

b renal failure.
c liver failure.

d water intoxication.

e Addison's disease.

96 **Pulmonary fibrosis**

a complicates bronchiectasis.
b results in an increase in pulmonary compliance.

c may supervene in chronic mitral valve disease.

d produces a restrictive defect in lung function tests.
e may occur following treatment with bleomycin.

97 **Tumours associated with a low serum potassium concentration include**

a chondrosarcoma.
b acoustic neuroma.
c carcinoid.

d villous papilloma of the rectum.
e phaeochromocytoma.

98 **P waves are absent from the ECG in**

a atrial fibrillation.
b ventricular tachycardia.

c massive pulmonary embolism.

d first degree heart block.

e nodal rhythm.

(Ch. 5, D)

a **False** Sodium retention secondary to aldosterone secretion is common in heart failure *(Ch. 3, D)*.
b **False** A low total body sodium does not accompany renal failure.
c **False** Sodium retention occurs because of impaired aldosterone metabolism.
d **False** Isolated water intoxication results from water retention in the presence of a normal total body sodium.
e **True** But serum cortisol concentration should be determined to make the diagnosis *(Ch. 8, D)*.

(Ch. 4, D)

a **True** 'Replacement' fibrosis is associated with bronchiectasis.
b **False** Increased stiffness of the lungs accounts for decreased compliance.
c **True** Pulmonary oedema becomes chronic, and interstitial fibrosis may follow.
d **True** Both FEV_1 and FVC are reduced.
e **True**

(Chs. 5 and 9, D)

a **False** Hypokalaemia is not a recognized feature.
b **False** This is not a recognized feature.
c **True** Diarrhoea is a feature of carcinoid syndrome, and electrolyte imbalance may occur.
d **True** This tumour is associated classically with potassium loss.
e **False** Phaeochromocytoma is a catecholamine-secreting tumour and is not associated with hypokalaemia.

(Ch. 3, D)

a **True** The fibrillary waves of atrial fibrillation do not constitute P waves.
b **True** In ventricular tachycardia, there is no time for automatic depolarization of the atria, and any atrial depolarization which occurs retrogradely is hidden in the ventricular waves.
c **False** P waves should not normally be absent with massive pulmonary embolism, unless asystole occurs.
d **False** In first degree heart block, the interval from the beginning of the P wave to the beginning of the R wave exceeds 0.2 s.
e **True** In nodal rhythm, ventricular depolarization is initiated at the atrioventricular node. It is impossible to detect P waves, as they occur synchronously with ventricular depolarization and are hidden in the QRS complex.

(Ch. 8, D)

99 **Tetany occurs in**
  a anoxia.
  b hypercalcaemia.
  c hypokalaemia.

  d alkalosis.

  e *Clostridium welchii* infection.

---

100 **An increased Pa_{CO_2} is found in the following:**
  a those living at altitude.
  b obstructive sleep apnoea.

  c early septicaemia.

  d acidosis from renal causes.

  e during infusion of bicarbonate.

(Ch. 8, D)

a **False** This is not a feature of anoxia.
b **False** Tetany is a feature of hypocalcaemia.
c **False** Hypokalaemia causes muscle flaccidity and cardiac arrhythmias *(Ch. 21, A & S)*.
d **True** Alkalosis reduces the serum concentration of ionized calcium; this causes tetany and a positive Chvostek's sign.
e **False** This is the causative organism of tetanus.

(Ch. 1, A & S)

a **False** Hyperventilation occurs during adaptation to altitude.
b **True** Hypoventilation occurs during episodes of obstructive sleep apnoea. This is common in the early postoperative period *(Ch. 23, A & S)*.
c **False** Early septicaemia is accompanied usually by hyperventilation *(Ch. 41, A & S)*.
d **False** Respiratory compensation for metabolic acidosis results in a decreased Pa_{CO_2}.
e **True** Bicarbonate forms an equilibrium with carbonic acid, which dissociates into carbon dioxide and water. A transient increase in Pa_{CO_2} occurs after infusion of bicarbonate.

4. Anaesthesia

1 A 70-year-old patient presents for gastrectomy. Preoperatively, Pa_{O_2} is 10.5 kPa on air. 15 min postoperatively, the patient is awake, breathing oxygen 3 l/min via nasal cannulae. Pa_{O_2} is 8 kPa; Pa_{CO_2} is 7 kPa. The following may be responsible for the abnormalities:

a reduced alveolar ventilation.

b diffusion hypoxia.

c decreased shunt.

d disturbed ventilation/perfusion ratio.

e depression of ventilation.

2 **The Bain system**

a is suitable for infants.

b is also a Mapleson C system.

c involves fresh gas flow through the outer tubing.

d if disconnected at the machine end causes increased dead space.

e requires a fresh gas flow rate of more than twice the minute volume with spontaneous ventilation in order to prevent rebreathing of carbon dioxide.

(Ch. 23, A & S)

a **True** The Pa_{CO_2} is elevated.
b **False** Diffusion hypoxia is transient and is treated effectively by oxygen therapy.
c **False** Shunting is likely to be increased.
d **True** This is present during anaesthesia and may persist into the early postoperative period.
e **True** The action of respiratory depressant drugs given intraoperatively may persist into the postoperative period.

(Ch. 16, A & S)

a **False** The system is not recommended for patients less than 25 kg in weight.
b **False** It is an example of a Mapleson D system.
c **False** The inner tube delivers fresh gas, and its attachment to the proximal end must be ensured before use of the system. The Lack breathing system (a coaxial form of the Mapleson A) has fresh gas flow through the outer tube.
d **True** The outer expiratory limb forms the extra dead space.
e **True** But it is more economical with IPPV (intermittent positive-pressure ventilation) – requiring only 70–100 ml/kg per min.

3   The Blease-Manley ventilator
a   is a minute volume divider.
b   is a constant flow generator.

c   is time-cycled.

d   is suitable for IPPV in the asthmatic.

e   may cause Rotameter inaccuracy.

---

4   A successful peribulbar block
a   is suggested by pupillary dilatation.

b   leads to ptosis.
c   needs the use of relatively small volumes of local anaesthetic.

d   would be more likely after the use of 5000 units of hyaluronidase.
e   would be more likely after the addition of 25 µg of adrenaline to the injectate.

---

5   In the axillary approach to brachial plexus block, the following are true:
a   The arm should be abducted to more than 90°.
b   The clavicle should be depressed.

c   The needle should pass alongside the axillary artery.

d   The block should be abandoned if the axillary artery is punctured.
e   Onset time is rapid.

(Ch. 16, A & S)

a **True** The fresh gas flow is divided into preset tidal volumes.
b **False** Constant flow cannot be generated by its relatively low working pressure. The descent of the inspiratory bellows under a preset weight provides a constant pressure.
c **True** Both between inspiration and expiration, and between expiration and inspiration. The timing is determined by the fresh gas flow rate and the tidal volume, and is changed if either parameter is altered.
d **False** High inflation pressures may be required in those with bronchospasm. A constant flow generator would be better.
e **True** This is due to back pressure in the machine and causes the Rotameter to under-read. Newer anaesthetic machines have a device to minimize this effect.

(Ch. 28, A & S)

a **False** This would be a manifestation of sympathetic stimulation. Dilatation of the pupil is usually achieved with locally applied mydriatric agents.
b **True**
c **False** Relative to retrobulbar or intraconal anaesthesia, large volumes are required – up to 10 ml of high-concentration local anaesthetic.
d **False** Hyaluronidase, 5 units per ml of local anaesthetic, is optimal. 5000 units would be a large overdose.
e **True** This is a concentration of 1:400 000, which improves the solidity and duration of the block.

(Ch. 25, A & S)

a **False** Abduction beyond 90° hinders performance of the block.
b **False** Asking the patient to touch the outside of his/her thigh is an aid to the supraclavicular approach.
c **True** The axillary artery is contained within the same neurovascular bundle as the plexus.
d **False** The local anaesthetic should be injected after passing through the artery and its posterior wall.
e **False** Onset time may be as long as 30–40 min.

6   The sciatic nerve
   a arises from the lumbar plexus.
   b might be blocked by a lateral approach through the thigh.

   c can be blocked with the femoral and lateral cutaneous nerve of the thigh in a 'three-in-one block' with a single injection.

   d block uses high doses of local anaesthetic, and systemic toxicity occurs commonly.

   e block leads to vasoconstriction in the area supplied.

---

7   Hypotension during subarachnoid block
   a may be due to preganglionic autonomic blockade.

   b should always be treated.

   c results from block of the dorsal roots.
   d is caused by stimulation of the vasomotor centre.

   e may be due to block of the nerves to the adrenal medulla.

---

8   The volume displacement of a strain gauge pressure transducer
   a indicates the amount of liquid needed to fill it.

   b depends on the volume of the chamber.
   c depends on the stiffness of the diaphragm.
   d depends on the frequency response of the system.
   e is pressure-dependent.

---

9   Halothane concentrations can be measured by
   a adsorption of vapour onto a crystal.

   b infrared absorption.
   c a Rayleigh refractometer.
   d changes in the elasticity of silicone rubber.

   e the Clark electrode.

(Ch. 25, A & S)

a **False** The sciatic nerve arises from the sacral plexus.
b **True** The supine approach through the lateral thigh is well described.
c **False** The 'three-in-one' block is designed for the lumbar plexus nerves – femoral, obturator and lateral cutaneous nerve of the thigh.
d **False** With the volume used normally, there is little risk of toxicity. However, there is a risk if other nerves are blocked; dilute local anaesthetic solutions and/or adrenaline are recommended to reduce the risk.
e **False** A successful block would result in vasodilatation.

(Ch. 25, A & S)

a **True** The dermatomal level of sympathetic blockade is higher than that of analgesia.
b **False** Treatment may not always be necessary; moderate hypotension may be beneficial and is tolerated well by most patients.
c **False** The dorsal roots carry afferent information only.
d **False** The brain stem vasomotor centre is unaffected unless the block is extremely high!
e **True** This is a contributory element in the genesis of hypotension.

(Ch. 20, A & S)

a **False** A continuous column of liquid is needed between the patient and the transducer, but this volume is unrelated to the volume displacement of the transducer.
b **False**
c **True** A stiff diaphragm is displaced to a lesser extent.
d **True** At resonant frequency, volume displacement is increased.
e **True**

(Ch. 20, A & S)

a **True** This changes the resonant frequency of a piezoelectric crystal. This is the principle used in the EMMA multigas analyser.
b **True**
c **True** This may be used to calibrate vaporizers.
d **True** This is a characteristic of halothane. It is the principle of the (now defunct) Dräger Narkotest.
e **False** This measures oxygen concentration.

10   Fuel cell analysers can be used for
a   oxygen analysis.

b CO_2 analysis.
c   measurement of oxygen percentage in inspired gas.

d   measurement of humidity.
e   breath-by-breath analysis of inspired gas.

---

11   Pressure gauges
a   may employ the Bourdon principle.
b   can be used to measure gas flow.

c   can regulate gas pressure.

d   can be used to measure temperature.

e   indicate absolute pressure.

---

12   During one-lung anaesthesia in the lateral position, Pa_{O_2} depends upon
a   inspired O_2.

b   cardiac output.

c   perfusion of the unventilated lung.

d   haematocrit.

e   mixed venous P_{O_2}.

(Ch. 20, A & S)

a **True** The galvanic cell generates current proportional to oxygen partial pressure.

b **False**

c **True** The partial pressure is measured. Back pressure influences the displayed concentration.

d **False** Humidity does not affect the reading of a fuel cell analyser.

e **False** The response time is too slow for breath-by-breath analysis.

(Ch. 15, A & S)

a **True** A coiled metal tube responds to differences in pressure.

b **True** Provided flow is laminar, the pressure gradient is directly proportional to the flow rate.

c **False** A pressure-reducing valve, which is more correctly termed a pressure-regulating valve, performs this task.

d **True** As the temperature of a gas is proportional to its pressure, this is theoretically possible; the pyrometer uses this principle.

e **False** Pressure gauges indicate gauge pressure, i.e. the pressure above ambient pressure.

(Ch. 38, A & S)

a **True** Because of intrapulmonary shunting, at least 40% inspired oxygen is required usually to achieve a normal Pa_{O_2}.

b **True** Low cardiac output may increase Pa_{O_2} if it causes reduced pulmonary artery pressure, resulting in decreased perfusion of the upper, unventilated lung. However, the arteriovenous oxygen content difference is increased by a reduction in cardiac output, and for a given shunt fraction, Pa_{O_2} is decreased.

c **True** Perfusion of the lungs varies with pulmonary artery pressure (see **b** above).

d **True** Decreased haematocrit may decrease oxygen delivery to the tissues, change atrioventricular (AV) content difference, and, for a given cardiac output and shunt fraction, affect Pa_{O_2}.

e **True**

13 **A 15-year-old child, whose brother died following an anaesthetic and having developed a high temperature, presents for elective surgery. The following should be performed in addition to normal investigations:**
   a   muscle biopsy.

   b   serum sodium concentration.
   c   creatinine phosphokinase concentration.
   d   cholinesterase concentration.

   e   urinalysis.

14 **The following are associated with increased intracolonic pressure:**
   a N_2O anaesthesia.
   b   morphine.

   c   neostigmine.
   d   adrenaline.

   e   an epidural block to T6.

15 **The following predispose to regurgitation of gastric contents into the pharynx:**
   a   hiatus hernia.

   b   raised intragastric pressure.

   c   induction in lithotomy position.

   d   head-down left lateral position.

   e   cricoid pressure.

16 **Junctional rhythm occurring during anaesthesia**
   a   is usually irregular.

   b   has an abnormal QRS complex.

   c   leads to a reduction in arterial pressure, requiring treatment.
   d   may be treated with i.v. atropine.

   e   is associated with the use of halothane.

a	**True**	The possibility of malignant hyperpyrexia should be entertained, and this test is specific.
b	**False**	
c	**False**	This test is insensitive.
d	**False**	**b**, **c** and **d** are unhelpful in the diagnosis of malignant hyperpyrexia.
e	**False**	This should be part of routine preoperative screening in any patient.

a	**True**	Nitrous oxide diffuses into air-filled body cavities *(Ch. 8, A & S)*.
b	**True**	Because of increase in non-propulsive smooth muscle activity of the gut *(Ch. 10, A & S)*.
c	**True**	This is mediated via activity in the parasympathetic end organ.
d	**False**	Sympathetic stimulation reduces splanchnic vascularity and activity *(Ch. 12, A & S)*.
e	**True**	The gut is contracted due to unopposed vagal activity *(Ch. 25, A & S)*.

a	**True**	Measures to reduce the acidity and volume of gastric contents should be taken in such patients.
b	**True**	Compression, such as that due to the gravid uterus (or obesity), causes this.
c	**True**	The gravitational effect of abdominal contents on the stomach is greater in the lithotomy position.
d	**False**	But if regurgitation occurs, aspiration is less likely in this position.
e	**False**	But pressure must be maintained to occlude the oesophagus.

a	**False**	The junctional node depolarizes in a regular manner but more slowly than the sinoatrial (SA) node.
b	**False**	QRS depolarization takes place via the normal pathway and is therefore of normal configuration.
c	**False**	But if hypovolaemia is present, arterial pressure may decrease.
d	**True**	When treatment is required, i.v. anticholinergic therapy is effective.
e	**True**	Halothane depresses automaticity of the SA node, and nodal arrhythmias are a common accompaniment of halothane anaesthesia.

17 **The following are generally accepted methods used to reduce suxamethonium muscle pain:**
   a deepening anaesthesia before use.

   b a prior dose of 100 µg/kg of vecuronium.

   c a prior small dose of suxamethonium.

   d concurrent use of morphine.

   e administration by infusion.

18 **During anaesthesia, signs of mismatched transfusion**
   a may include raised arterial pressure.
   b may be obscured.

   c include oozing.

   d include haematuria.
   e include conjunctival petechiae.

19 **During prolonged operations, core temperature can be monitored accurately at the**
   a tympanic membrane.
   b lower third of oesophagus.
   c muscle in thigh.

   d nasopharynx.
   e pulmonary vein.

(Ch. 23, A & S)

a	**False**	Deep anaesthesia before administration of suxamethonium has not been shown to reduce suxamethonium-related muscle pains.
b	**False**	This is a normal paralysing dose. The dose of non-depolarizing muscle relaxant needed to reduce suxamethonium pain is small – approximately one tenth of that used to establish neuromuscular block.
c	**True**	The administration of a small dose of suxamethonium (0.1 mg/kg) has been described as reducing the pain due to the subsequent administration of suxamethonium.
d	**False**	Morphine and other opioids have not been shown to reduce suxamethonium muscle pain.
e	**True**	The administration of suxamethonium by infusion is generally accepted as reducing the incidence of suxamethonium pain.

(Ch. 6, A & S)

a	**False**	Hypotension is usual.
b	**True**	General anaesthesia may mask the early signs of any transfusion reaction.
c	**True**	This may be an early sign of mismatched transfusion and is due to consumption coagulopathy.
d	**True**	Due to red cell destruction.
e	**False**	This is a sign typical of fat embolus.

(Ch. 20, A & S)

a	**True**	This is used as an index of brain temperature.
b	**True**	This reflects heart temperature.
c	**False**	Muscle temperature may be influenced by the state of the peripheral circulation.
d	**True**	The probe must be in contact with the pharyngeal mucosa.
e	**False**	The pulmonary vein is not cannulated for monitoring purposes.

20   The following are true of compressed medical gases:

a   Oxygen is normally stored at a pressure of 800 kPa.

b   Nitrous oxide is stored in cylinders at a pressure of 400 kPa.

c   Nitrous oxide cylinders are filled to 90% of their volume with liquid by the manufacturers.

d   They are stored in cylinders of molybdenum steel.

e   The amount of oxygen in a cylinder is determined by weighing.

21   During anaesthesia, a patient with Parkinson's disease treated with levodopa should not receive

a   enflurane.
b   fentanyl.
c   morphine.
d   droperidol.

e   nitrous oxide.

22   Oliguria postoperatively is associated with

a   methoxyflurane anaesthesia.
b   low cardiac output.

c   hypothermia.
d   hypoglycaemia.
e   hypovolaemia.

23   The following give an early and reliable indication of the occurrence of air embolism:

a   ECG.
b   BP monitoring.
c   end-tidal CO_2.

d   Doppler ultrasound.
e   oesophageal auscultation.

(Ch. 16, A & S)

a	**False**	Oxygen may be stored safely at this pressure, but the usual pressure of a full oxygen cylinder is 13.7 MPa; the pressure in pipeline delivery systems is 400 kPa.
b	**False**	Nitrous oxide can be stored at 400 kPa, the pipeline pressure. However, the pressure in a full nitrous oxide cylinder is 4.4 MPa.
c	**True**	The normal 'filling ratio' of a nitrous oxide cylinder is 0.67 – this is related to the weight of nitrous oxide/weight of water needed to fill the cylinder. If it was full, the liquid would expand as the temperature rises above the critical temperature, with a catastrophic increase in pressure *(Ch. 15, A & S)*.
d	**True**	These cylinders offer an acceptable compromise between strength and weight.
e	**False**	Strictly, the amount of oxygen in a cylinder can be determined by weighing and by reference to the tare (empty weight) of the cylinder. However, as the oxygen is present as compressed gas, the change in weight is very small as the cylinder empties and this method is not of practical value.

(Ch. 14, D)

a	**False**	Enflurane is not contraindicated.
b	**False**	There is no contraindication to the use of fentanyl.
c	**False**	Morphine is not contraindicated.
d	**True**	Extrapyramidal side-effects of droperidol are commonly observed. It is a DOPA antagonist *(Ch. 4, BNF)*.
e	**False**	Nitrous oxide is not contraindicated.

(Ch. 23, A & S)

a	**False**	Methoxyflurane toxicity is associated with polyuria.
b	**True**	Low cardiac output results in decreased renal blood flow. Acute tubular necrosis may occur.
c	**False**	Hypothermia *per se* would not lead to oliguria.
d	**False**	Oliguria would not result from hypoglycaemia.
e	**True**	Hypovolaemia leads to decreased cardiac output and increased secretion of antidiuretic hormone (ADH).

(Chs. 22 and 37, A & S)

a	**False**	ECG changes are a very late sign.
b	**False**	This is not a reliable indicator of air embolism.
c	**True**	End-tidal carbon dioxide concentration decreases due to decreased perfusion of alveoli.
d	**True**	This is an extremely sensitive method of detection of air emboli.
e	**False**	The classical 'mill-wheel' murmur is heard late, and only with a large volume of air.

24 **With regard to transplacental passage of drugs**
a the placenta is an effective barrier.
b fetal bradycardia may occur after epidural injection of local anaesthetics.

c highly protein-bound drugs are transferred less readily.

d amide-linked local anaesthetic drugs should be avoided.

e fetal bradycardia is related directly to fetal blood concentration of local anaesthetic.

---

25 **During lumbar epidural anaesthesia for Caesarean section**
a never give more than 20 ml of 0.5% bupivacaine.

b the block must extend from T5 to S1.

c syntocinon rather than ergometrine should be used.
d a paracervical block must also be performed.
e the circulation should be preloaded with Hartmann's solution.

---

26 **You are asked to provide anaesthesia for a patient with a breech delivery when difficulty is being experienced with the fetal head. The following are acceptable techniques:**
a spinal or subarachnoid block.

b epidural or extradural block.
c halothane.

d thiopentone, suxamethonium, rapid-sequence tracheal intubation.
e ketamine.

(Chs. 5 and 32, A & S)

a	**False**	Lipid-soluble drugs cross the placenta readily.
b	**True**	Toxic concentrations cross the placenta. Acceptable maternal concentrations may produce much larger fetal concentrations because of the relatively acid state of the fetal environment.
c	**False**	The free drug concentration determines the amount of placental transfer.
d	**False**	Bupivacaine and lignocaine are both acceptable agents in obstetric analgesia.
e	**True**	

(Ch. 32, A & S; Ch. 15, BNF)

a	**False**	The maximum recommended dose of bupivacaine 0.5% is 20 ml. However, a single dose of up to 150 mg of bupivacaine (30 ml of 0.5% solution) is permissible for appropriate patients.
b	**False**	A block to S5 is necessary for adequate analgesia for Caesarean section.
c	**True**	Syntocinon provokes less nausea than does ergometrine.
d	**False**	Properly conducted epidural block is sufficient.
e	**True**	Up to 1000 ml of Hartmann's solution has been recommended as a preload for epidural Caesarean sections, but colloid solutions may be preferable. More recent work has suggested that preloading with 500 ml of crystalloid is sufficient.

(Ch. 32, A & S)

a	**True**	The anaesthetist should be experienced at subarachnoid techniques; this would be inappropriate for anaesthetists who are new to obstetric anaesthesia.
b	**False**	Onset time would be much too long.
c	**False**	Unless the anaesthetist is familiar with the use of halothane in obstetric practice, this is inappropriate.
d	**True**	A rapid-sequence induction with a familiar technique is indicated.
e	**True**	Ketamine may be indicated in a domiciliary situation, but would not be the technique of first choice in hospital.

27   Coeliac plexus block
a   may relieve abdominal visceral pain.
b   may relieve pain of acute pancreatitis.

c   cannot be performed without X-ray control.

d   may cause profound hypotension.
e   requires the tip of the needle to lie at the level of L1.

28   Block of the trigeminal ganglion is associated with anaesthesia of
a   alae nasi.

b   lower lip.
c   angle of mandible.

d   soft palate.
e   eardrum.

29   If 50% nitrous oxide is inhaled for 3 days
a   the lymphocyte count falls.

b   methionine synthetase activity is reduced.
c   megaloblastic bone marrow changes occur.
d B_{12}-deficiency anaemia develops.

e   peripheral neuropathy develops.

30   Helium
a   has a viscosity similar to that of oxygen.

b   is supplied in liquid form in brown cylinders.

c   inhalation causes voice changes.
d   is used to decrease the work of breathing in bronchospasm.

e   supports combustion.

(Ch. 42, A & S)

a True The coeliac plexus innervates the abdominal viscera.
b True But is employed usually for chronic pain relief in association with pancreatic carcinoma.
c False This is possible, but the technique is more likely to be successful when an image intensifier is used. X-ray control is now regarded as mandatory.
d True Due to sympathetic blockade.
e True This is where the coeliac plexus lies.

(Chs. 4 and 42, A & S)

a True The second division of the trigeminal nerve supplies the nasal area.
b True The third division of the trigeminal nerve supplies this region.
c False The angle of the mandible is supplied by the anterior rami of spinal nerves C2–3.
d False This is supplied by the glossopharyngeal nerve.
e True The auriculotemporal nerve, a branch of the third division of the trigeminal, supplies the tympanic membrane.

(Ch. 8, A & S)

a True Nitrous oxide exhibits a depressant effect on methionine synthetase activity and folic acid metabolism, and impairs synthesis of DNA. After prolonged inhalation, agranulocytosis and bone marrow aplasia may result.
b True See **a** above.
c True See **a** above.
d False Although there are megaloblastic changes, these are not attributable to vitamin B_{12} deficiency, nor would this type of anaemia develop in 3 days.
e False Although occupational exposure can lead to a myeloneuropathy, this has not been reported in acute exposure.

a True It may be given accurately at low flows through an oxygen rotameter. Its density is one-eighth that of oxygen *(Ch. 15, A & S)*.
b False Helium cylinders contain gaseous helium at room temperature *(Ch. 16, A & S)*.
c True Its low density causes a change in the timbre of the voice.
d False Helium does not relieve lower airway obstruction. However, it is used commonly as a temporary expedient in upper airway obstruction, when flow is turbulent.
e False Helium is non-flammable and does not support combustion.

31 The following are appropriate statements about premedication:

a   atropine is used to induce sedation.

b   lorazepam causes anxiolysis.

c   hyoscine is an anticholinergic.

d   papaveretum relieves anxiety.

e   phenothiazines are anticholinergics.

32 Concerning preoperative assessment

a   haemoglobin concentration should be available for all patients undergoing elective surgery.

b   a chest X-ray is not required routinely in patients less than 60 years of age.

c   a patient with incapacitating disease which constantly threatens life is in ASA grade IV.

d   a healthy patient with only mild systemic disease is classed as ASA grade II.

e   the mortality rate of patients in ASA grade IV approaches 12%.

33 Halothane hepatotoxicity is associated with

a   the elderly.

b   obesity.

c   prolonged anaesthesia.

d   history of cholecystitis.

e   oxidative enzymatic degradation.

(Ch. 18, A & S)

a **False** Atropine may cause central stimulation. Hyoscine is more sedative.

b **True** Benzodiazepines possess anxiolytic actions in doses unlikely to produce sedation.

c **True** Hyoscine is an anticholinergic but should be avoided in the elderly because of dysphoria and restlessness.

d **False** Although good sedatives, opioids have poor anxiolytic actions.

e **True** Phenothiazines possess atropine-like actions.

(Ch. 18, A & S)

a **False** Measurement of haemoglobin is suggested for all patients undergoing major surgery, males over 50 years of age, all females, and when indicated by the presence of systemic disease.

b **True** But the presence of cardiac or respiratory disease or the likelihood of thoracic surgery indicates the need for preoperative chest X-ray.

c **True**

d **True**

e **False** The mortality rate for ASA grade IV patients is quoted as 7.8%; for ASA grade V, the figure is 9.4%.

(Ch. 8, A & S)

a **False** Hepatotoxicity with halothane has been reported in all adult age groups, and none predominates.

b **True** Obese patients seem to retain halothane longer than thinner ones, and this seems to predispose to halothane hepatotoxicity.

c **False** A single prolonged anaesthetic is not associated particularly with halothane hepatotoxicity.

d **False** There is no association between cholecystitis and halothane hepatotoxicity.

e **False** The mechanism of hepatotoxicity is associated with reductive enzyme pathways.

34 Suxamethonium is contraindicated in

a   acute intermittent porphyria.

b   congestive cardiac failure.

c   chronic renal failure controlled with dialysis.

d   myotonia dystrophica.

e   a patient who has been paraplegic for 1 year.

35 During anaesthesia for laparotomy in a patient with glomerulonephritis

a   mannitol 1.5 g/kg should be given.

b   ibuprofen should be avoided for postoperative pain relief, as it decreases renal blood flow.

c   halothane should be avoided because it is nephrotoxic.

d   a sympathomimetic should be given to increase glomerular filtration rate (GFR).

e   alteration in plasma protein concentrations may affect neuromuscular blocking activity.

36 Postoperative pain in adults may be treated appropriately with

a   morphine, by infusion to achieve a plasma concentration of 8 ng/ml.

b   i.m. papaveretum in a dose of 15.4 mg, 4-hourly for a 70 kg adult.

c   patient-controlled analgesia with buprenorphine.

d   oral sustained-release preparations of morphine.

e   bilateral intercostal blocks for upper abdominal surgery.

(Chs. 11 and 40, A & S)

a **False** Suxamethonium is not contraindicated in acute intermittent porphyria.
b **False** This is not a contraindication.
c **False** However, dialysis may lead to a marked reduction in plasma cholinesterase activity – and some prolongation of neuromuscular blockade.
d **True** Suxamethonium has been associated with intense muscle rigidity in the presence of myotonia dystrophica.
e **False** But suxamethonium is contraindicated in early paraplegia. Administration in the presence of muscular denervation can result in profound hyperkalaemia afterwards.

(Ch. 40, A & S)

a **False** Mannitol is not indicated in this condition.
b **True** Ibuprofen (and other NSAIDs) inhibits vasodilator prostaglandin secretion. Reduction in glomerular blood flow and sodium excretion may be critical; its use should be restricted in high-risk patients.
c **False** Halothane is not nephrotoxic and is not contraindicated.
d **False** Sympathomimetic agents can cause a reduction in renal blood flow and consequently GFR *(Ch. 12, A & S)*.
e **True** The albumin:globulin ratio is reversed, and protein binding of neuromuscular agents is altered.

(Ch. 24, A & S)

a **False** The minimum effective analgesic concentration (MEAC) for morphine infusions is about twice this value (12–24 ng/ml).
b **True** But conventional i.m. use carries several disadvantages.
c **False** Buprenorphine is a partial agonist opioid analgesic. It is usually used sublingually.
d **False** There is a reduction in the rate of gastric emptying postoperatively. This may lead to accumulation in the stomach, followed by unpredictably delayed absorption or 'dumping'.
e **False** Although unilateral intercostal blockade is recommended after 'open' cholecystectomy through a subcostal incision, bilateral block is not recommended because of the risk of pneumothorax.

37 The management of chronic (intractable) pain in a young adult may include the following:

a frequent i.m. injection of morphine.

b oral antidepressants.

c radiofrequency ablative lesions.

d facial nerve blockade for unilateral facial pain.

e coeliac plexus block for intra-abdominal malignancy.

---

38 Hazards in the operating theatre are minimized if

a a theatre temperature of 22–24°C is combined with a relative humidity of 50%.

b only non-isolated electrical equipment is used.

c volatile agent concentration in the atmosphere is limited to 100 p.p.m. (parts per million) by the use of scavenging apparatus.

d needles are never resheathed when a patient with hepatitis B is undergoing anaesthesia.

e reusable equipment is soaked in 2% glutaraldehyde for 3 h following use on a patient with AIDS.

---

39 Cardiac arrhythmias during halothane anaesthesia

a are less frequent during light anaesthesia.

b are more frequent during hypercapnia.

c can be terminated using a beta-blocker.

d are more frequent in the presence of hyperkalaemia.

e may result in a reduction of blood pressure.

(Ch. 42, A & S)

a **False** Injections should be avoided for long-term therapy. Oral or rectal administration is preferred.

b **True** Analgesic activity of opioids may be enhanced by concurrent administration of a tricyclic antidepressant.

c **True** Temperatures of above 50°C are achieved at the tip of the probe. These lesions are commonly performed and are quite specific.

d **False** The facial nerve is motor to the facial muscles. Trigeminal nerve blockade may be appropriate treatment for facial pain.

e **True** Pain arising as a result of pancreatic neoplasia responds to the injection of alcohol into the coeliac plexus.

(Ch. 17, A & S)

a **True** Patients are at risk of hypothermia at an ambient temperature below 21°C. Neonatal surgery demands higher ambient temperatures (Ch. 33, A & S).

b **False** All modern monitoring equipment (and other equipment such as that for diathermy) is 'isolated' by means of an isolating transformer.

c **False** The recommended maximum concentration of volatile agents in the theatre environment in the UK by HSE (the Health and Safety Executive) is 10 p.p.m. (halothane) – 50 p.p.m. (isoflurane and enflurane). In the US by NIOSH (National Institute of Occupational Safety and Hygiene) it is much lower – 2 p.p.m. However, hazards to theatre staff as a result of occupational exposure to pollutants may have been exaggerated.

d **True** Resheathing of needles is not recommended after use on any patient.

e **True** Thorough washing before immersion is recommended. Disposable equipment should be used whenever possible.

(Ch. 8, A & S)

a **False** They are more frequent during light anaesthesia.

b **True** Hypercapnia provokes sympatho-adrenal activity.

c **True** But beta-blockers must be used with caution in the presence of halothane – excessive doses may cause bradycardia and profound hypotension.

d **True** Ventricular arrhythmias arise with hyperkalaemia.

e **True** But usually there is little effect.

40 Nitrous oxide

a decreases the response of ventilation to hypercapnia.

b is slightly less soluble than nitrogen in blood.

c may be associated with postoperative hearing loss.

d may be associated with bone marrow dysplasia after prolonged administration.

e does not support combustion.

---

41 The pressure in a half-filled nitrous oxide cylinder depends upon
a the percentage of liquid N_2O present.
b the ambient temperature.
c the saturated vapour pressure of N_2O.

d the molecular weight of N_2O.
e the pseudo-critical temperature.

---

42 The Mapleson A breathing system

a is a partial rebreathing system.

b requires a fresh gas flow (FGF) rate of 2 × minute volume to prevent rebreathing of alveolar gas during spontaneous ventilation.
c requires a FGF rate of 3 × minute volume to prevent rebreathing of alveolar gas during spontaneous ventilation.
d requires 100 ml/kg FGF during IPPV.
e forms the basis of the Lack system.

---

43 Control of intraocular pressure (IOP) during induction of anaesthesia
a concerns the same factors as those controlling intracranial pressure.
b can be achieved safely with ketamine.
c may contraindicate the need for suxamethonium in the emergency patient with a penetrating eye injury.

d is important to minimize loss of vitreous when a penetrating eye injury is present.
e is necessary during squint surgery.

(Ch. 8, A & S)

a True There is mild depression of the response of ventilation to carbon dioxide.

b False The blood/gas solubility coefficient of nitrous oxide is 0.47, and that of nitrogen 0.015 *(Appendix II, A & S)*.

c True Caused by diffusion into the middle ear, with a consequent increase in pressure.

d True This results from suppression of vitamin B_{12} and methionine synthetase activity. This can occur after short anaesthesia in critically ill patients.

e False Nitrous oxide supports combustion, although it is not flammable.

(Ch. 15, A & S)

a False This does not influence the pressure in the cylinder.

b True Temperature influences the saturated vapour pressure.

c True It is the only property of the agent which determines pressure in the cylinder.

d False

e False This relates to pre-mixed nitrous oxide and oxygen – Entonox. It is the temperature (–7°C) at which Entonox separates into its constituent parts.

(Ch. 16, A & S)

a True However, when the FGF rate equals alveolar minute ventilation, only dead space gas is rebreathed.

b False See **a** above *(Appendix X, A & S)*.

c False See **a** above *(Appendix X, A & S)*.

d False Usually at least 2.5–3 times the minute volume is required.

e True The Lack system is a coaxial form of the Mapleson A system.

(Ch. 28, A & S)

a True Pa_{CO_2} is a major determinant of IOP. Other factors include Pa_{O_2}, posture and venous drainage.

b False Ketamine increases IOP.

c False Suxamethonium is indicated during rapid-sequence induction when difficulty is anticipated with tracheal intubation in an unfasted patient.

d True Vitreous prolapse may occur with acute increases in IOP.

e False Extraocular surgery may be performed under any suitable anaesthetic technique.

44 The Mark 5 TEC vaporizer
a is a temperature-compensated vaporizer.
b should be used with a minimum fresh gas flow rate of 3 l/min.
c should be used with a minimum fresh gas flow rate of 2 l/min.
d is affected by back pressure when fresh gas flow rate is greater than 2 l/min.
e can be used as a drawover vaporizer.

45 Postoperative vomiting
a is always accompanied by nausea.
b is less frequent when hyoscine is given as part of premedication.
c increases the risk of postoperative pulmonary atelectasis.
d is more likely if opioid analgesics are given postoperatively.
e is more common in men than in women.

46 The following breathing systems require a fresh gas flow rate greater than the patient's minute volume to prevent rebreathing of carbon dioxide during spontaneous ventilation:
a Magill attachment.
b Mapleson E.
c Lack.
d circle system with CO_2 absorption.
e Mapleson C.

47 A Wright respirometer may be used alone to measure
a tidal volume (V_T).
b peak flow rate (PEFR).
c anatomical dead space ($V_{D(ANAT)}$).
d minute volume.
e functional residual capacity (FRC).

(Chs. 15 and 17, A & S)

a **True** The mechanism is a bimetallic strip.
b **False** The Mark 5 is accurate down to a FGF rate of less than 1 l/min.
c **False** See **b** above.
d **False** The Mark 5 Fluotec is unaffected by back pressure.

e **False** The internal resistance is too high for it to be used in this way.

(Ch. 23, A & S)

a **False** Vomiting is not invariably associated with nausea.
b **True** Hyoscine possesses anticholinergic actions, which confer an antiemetic action.
c **True** Secondary to the risk of aspiration.
d **True** Opioid analgesics have an emetic action.
e **False** It tends to be more common in women.

(Ch. 16 and Appendix X, A & S)

a **False** FGF of approximately the alveolar minute volume ensures efficient carbon dioxide elimination.
b **True** 2.5–3 × minute volume is required.
c **False** The Lack system is a coaxial form of the Magill (Mapleson A) system.
d **False** A FGF rate of less than 1 l/min may be used.
e **True** It is an inefficient breathing system, and requires a fresh gas flow rate of 2.5 × minute volume.

(Ch. 20, A & S)

a **True** But it is inaccurate at very high or very low tidal volumes.
b **False** Used in this way, damage to the vanes of the respirometer may result.
c **False** Measurement of carbon dioxide concentration is required as well as volume.
d **False** A stopwatch will be required!
e **False** FRC is measured by the helium dilution method.

48 **Central cyanosis in a patient in the immediate postanaesthetic recovery period may be due to**

a shivering.

b replacement of blood by crystalloid fluid.

c malignant hyperthermia.
d diffusion hypoxia.

e low cardiac output.

49 **The following occur frequently in the early postoperative period:**
a hypertension.

b hypocalcaemia.

c decreased lipolysis.

d shivering.

e suxamethonium pains.

50 **Heat loss during surgery can be minimized by**
a maintaining environmental temperature at 20°C.

b the use of a polythene 'bubble-wrap' blanket intraoperatively.

c administration of i.v. fluids via central lines.
d humidification of inspired gases.

e small doses of phenothiazines.

(Ch. 23, A & S)

a **True** Shivering increases oxygen demand. Desaturation of arterial blood may result unless supplemental oxygen is supplied.
b **False** With haemodilution, insufficient desaturated haemoglobin may be present for cyanosis to be detected.
c **True** Malignant hyperthermia may arise in the postoperative period.
d **True** Oxygen should be given in the immediate postoperative period to all patients who have been breathing a nitrous oxide/oxygen mixture.
e **True** Because of resultant increased venous admixture.

(Ch. 23, A & S)

a **True** This may occur as a manifestation of pain, hypoxaemia, hypercapnia, etc.
b **False** But reduction in ionized calcium (Ca^{++}) may occur transiently with hyperventilation.
c **False** The catabolic response to surgery results usually in increased lipolysis.
d **True** Commonly after volatile agents. Supplementary oxygen should be administered.
e **False** The incidence is 50% in those receiving the drug, but the onset is usually related to ambulation and would not be seen early.

(Ch. 22, A & S)

a **False** The thermoneutral environmental temperature for an unclothed adult is 27°C. Theatre temperature is usually maintained at about 22°C.
b **True** Covering exposed surfaces with 'bubble wrap' minimizes heat loss.
c **False** Warming of i.v. fluids is recommended to minimize heat loss.
d **True** Inhalation of cold dry gases necessitates heating and humidification by the respiratory tract. Humidification of inspired gases reduces loss of latent heat through vaporization.
e **False** Small doses of phenothiazines act as vasodilators and reduce core temperature.

51 Ketamine hallucinations are less troublesome
a in children.
b with diazepam premedication.

c with an opioid premedication.

d in outpatients.

e during recovery in quiet surroundings.

52 Waste gas scavenging systems
a present significantly increased resistance to expiration.

b may employ activated charcoal.
c should incorporate an active disposal system.

d employ connectors of 19 mm diameter to avoid cross-connections.

e employ negative pressure valves.

53 Concerning total i.v. anaesthesia
a ketamine can be employed.

b it can be employed safely in the presence of upper airway obstruction.
c it requires a loading dose at induction.

d the depth of anaesthesia is judged by eye signs.

e nitrous oxide/oxygen cannot be used in conjunction.

(Ch. 9, A & S)

a **False** But children may not report hallucinations.
b **True** Diazepam and lorazepam have been advocated for premedication to reduce the emergence phenomena associated with ketamine.
c **True** Although opioids may themselves cause dysphoric reactions, they are reported to reduce emergence delirium and hallucinations with ketamine.
d **False** Ketamine is generally considered to be an unsuitable agent for outpatient anaesthesia.
e **True** It is recommended that patients who have received ketamine should be nursed in quiet surroundings consistent with normal observation of airway and vital signs.

(Ch. 16, A & S)

a **False** Resistance to expiration is not normally increased. Care should be exercised in positioning tubing to avoid accidental compression.
b **True** Activated charcoal may be employed to adsorb volatile agents.
c **False** Passive and active systems are available. An active system is not always necessary.
d **False** Connectors are of 30 mm diameter to avoid inadvertent connection to anaesthetic delivery systems.
e **True** Negative pressure relief valves prevent transmission of negative pressure to the system.

a **True** Ketamine can be used as the sole anaesthetic agent, but its use must be preceded by the injection of atropine (Ch. 9, A & S).
b **False** Airway patency must be ensured before the use of any intravenous anaesthetic agent.
c **True** In order rapidly to achieve the steady state condition at which infusion rate is equal to elimination rate, a loading dose is given (Ch. 7, A & S).
d **False** Eye signs originally described by Guedel are not a reliable monitor of non-inhalational anaesthesia (Ch. 19, A & S).
e **True** Although nitrous oxide can be used to supplement intravenous anaesthesia, the technique cannot be *total* intravenous anaesthesia.

54 **Inguinal herniorrhaphy can be performed under the following types of anaesthesia:**
a paravertebral block at T10–12.
b epidural block using 20 ml lignocaine 1% at L3–4.
c saddle block.

d caudal block with 3 ml of ropivacaine 0.5%.

e subarachnoid block using 3 ml of heavy bupivacaine 0.5%.

---

55 **Hypertension in the postoperative period is commonly due to**
a hypocapnia.
b phaeochromocytoma.

c full bladder.

d surgical pain.

e volatile anaesthetic agents.

---

56 **A young healthy adult presents for thyroidectomy:**
a preoperative thyroid function testing is indicated.
b thoracic inlet X-ray examination is indicated preoperatively.

c preoperative beta-blockers may be indicated.

d Lugol's iodine should be given preoperatively to reduce vascularity.
e postoperative respiratory obstruction may occur due to tracheal collapse.

(Ch. 25, A & S)

a	**False**	Injection should be performed at T11, T12, L1 and L2.
b	**True**	This is an acceptable technique for inguinal herniorrhaphy.
c	**False**	A saddle block affects only the lower sacral segments, which form a ring around the anus. This is an unsuitable block for herniorrhaphy.
d	**False**	3 ml local anaesthetic injected into the caudal space produces minimal spread of anaesthesia.
e	**True**	This should produce an adequate block for inguinal herniorrhaphy.

(Ch. 23, A & S)

a	**False**	Hypocapnia alone does not produce hypertension.
b	**False**	Phaeochromocytoma is a very rare cause of hypertension in the postoperative period.
c	**True**	A full bladder can be very distressing and can result in an increase in arterial pressure.
d	**True**	Surgical pain may have either a hyper- or a hypotensive effect, and should be corrected before other causes of deranged arterial pressure are investigated.
e	**False**	All volatile anaesthetic agents depress the cardiovascular system, and do not cause hypertension in the postoperative period.

(Ch. 40, A & S; Ch. 8, D)

a	**True**	Hyperthyroidism must be corrected before elective surgery.
b	**False**	If the possibility of retrosternal spread of tumour is present or if tracheal compression is suspected, neck and thoracic inlet X-ray examination should be requested.
c	**True**	Control of symptoms may be achieved by preoperative oral treatment with beta-blockers. Treatment should continue into the postoperative period.
d	**False**	Potassium iodide t.i.d. has superseded the use of Lugol's iodine solution.
e	**True**	Pressure exerted by a goitre may erode the tracheal cartilage and result in loss of support. Such patients present with airway obstruction on inspiration *(Ch. 23, A & S)*.

57 **The following techniques are appropriate during reduction of dislocation of the shoulder:**
a   Bier's block.

b   axillary brachial plexus block.

c   interscalene block.

d   general anaesthesia.
e   diazepam sedation.

---

58 **Static electricity**
a   can cause a hypoxic mixture to be given via the Rotameters.

b   is produced by two non-conducting surfaces.

c   is removed by wetting the surfaces.

d   is reduced by ionizing radiation.

e   is reduced by the use of a conducting breathing system.

---

59 **Inhalational induction may be used in the following circumstances:**
a   acute epiglottitis.

b   a patient with a full stomach.

c   bronchopleural fistula.

d   tension pneumothorax.

e   maxillary fracture.

(Ch. 25, A & S)

a **False** A Bier's block (IVRA – intravenous regional anaesthesia) does not anaesthetize the shoulder as the tourniquet is placed on the upper arm!

b **False** This would anaesthetize the lower arm well, but not the shoulder.

c **True** A brachial plexus block, using the interscalene approach, could be used to reduce a dislocated shoulder but is not performed commonly in this situation.

d **True** General anaesthesia can be used.

e **False** Diazepam is required in anaesthetic doses for reduction of a dislocated shoulder, and other techniques are more appropriate.

(Chs. 15 and 16, A & S)

a **True** Modern Rotameters incorporate antistatic devices, but static electricity can cause the bobbins to stick to the side of the tube and provide a false indication of flow.

b **True** It is necessary for two non-conducting surfaces to allow the build-up of charge.

c **True** Wetting the surface decreases insulation and increases conductivity.

d **False** The static charge on a surface may be increased by ionizing radiation, due to displacement of electrons.

e **True** Although flammable anaesthetic agents are rarely used, the presence of the yellow stripe on black rubber indicates conductivity of the breathing system, and this minimizes the build-up of static charge.

(Ch. 19, A & S)

a **True** This is the method of choice. Intravenous injection before anaesthesia may precipitate complete airway obstruction *(Ch. 33, A & S)*.

b **False** Rapid-sequence intravenous induction is mandatory in such cases *(Ch. 31, A & S)*.

c **True** It is necessary to avoid contamination of the 'good' lung and avoid producing a pneumothorax with IPPV. Inhalational induction in the sitting position is a useful option before insertion of a double-lumen tube *(Ch. 38, A & S)*.

d **False** Anaesthesia should not be given in the presence of a tension pneumothorax. Nitrous oxide increases the pressure in a pneumothorax. An underwater-seal drain is mandatory before anaesthesia *(Ch. 22, A & S)*.

e **False** The potential for bleeding in the upper airway precludes the use of inhalational induction. Rapid-sequence induction with suction apparatus immediately to hand is the method of choice.

60 **Nasotracheal intubation is contraindicated in the following:**
a fractured base of skull.

b exodontia.

c a patient with a bleeding diathesis.

d Guillain–Barré syndrome.

e uncomplicated myocardial infarction.

---

61 **The following structures are traversed during midline lumbar epidural puncture:**
a ligamentum flavum.

b supraspinous ligament.
c ligamentum denticulum.

d posterior longitudinal ligament.

e stratum spinosum.

---

62 **The following disinfectants are effective decontaminants in a breathing system:**
a ethylene oxide.

b chlorhexidine hydrochloride in spirit.

c chlorhexidine hydrochloride in water.

d glutaraldehyde for 3 h.
e cetrimide solution BPC (1%).

a **True** Nasal haemorrhage may result and the potential for introduction of infection exists.
b **False** A nasal tube permits access to the mouth during dental surgery and allows better positioning of a throat pack *(Ch. 34, A & S)*.
c **True** Haemorrhage following trauma to the nasopharyngeal mucosa is a complication of nasal intubation *(Ch. 19, A & S)*.
d **False** Long-term tracheal intubation may be required and the nasal route carries some advantages in this respect *(Chs. 19 and 40, A & S)*.
e **False** When tracheal intubation is required, there is no contraindication to the use of the nasal route.

(Ch. 25, A & S)

a **True** The epidural needle passes in turn through the supraspinous ligament, interspinous ligament and the ligamentum flavum.
b **True** See **a** above.
c **False** The ligamentum denticulum lies within the subarachnoid space and is attached to the spinal cord.
d **False** The posterior longitudinal ligament is not traversed during lumbar epidural puncture.
e **True** This is part of the epidermis of the skin, which is traversed during epidural puncture.

(Ch. 17, A & S)

a **True** The gas may be explosive in air and is commonly used in combination with carbon dioxide.
b **False** Chlorhexidine in alcohol is used as a skin preparation preoperatively.
c **False** Aqueous chlorhexidine may be used for bladder irrigation and catheter lubrication.
d **True** After prior washing in soap and water.
e **False** Cetrimide, which also has detergent properties, is used predominantly for skin disinfection *(Ch. 13, BNF)*.

63 **The following are common causes of hypotension during anaesthesia:**

a hypercapnia.
b hypovolaemia.

c vecuronium.

d rocuronium.

e isoflurane.

---

64 **Nitrous oxide**

a is taken up rapidly and anaesthesia is rapidly attained.

b cylinders contain small amounts of nitric oxide and nitrogen dioxide.

c can give rise to bone marrow depression.
d can give rise to methaemoglobinaemia after prolonged administration.
e lowers the MAC of a concurrently administered agent.

---

65 **When administering anaesthesia to a patient suspected of being susceptible to malignant hyperpyrexia (MHS)**

a Premedication with morphine and atropine should be used.
b Vecuronium is a good choice of muscle relaxant.
c Nitrous oxide should be avoided.
d Dantrolene should be immediately available.

e Total i.v. anaesthesia (TIVA) with propofol is a safe technique.

(Ch. 22, A & S)

a	**False**	Hypercapnia leads to myocardial stimulation and hypertension.
b	**True**	Hypovolaemia due to either preoperative fluid loss or surgical blood loss results in hypotension.
c	**False**	Vecuronium has no significant actions on the cardiovascular system *(Ch. 11, A & S)*.
d	**False**	Rocuronium can cause a slight tachycardia. Its use is unlikely to result in hypotension *(Ch. 11, A & S)*.
e	**True**	Isoflurane causes peripheral vasodilatation and hypotension, with a reactive tachycardia *(Ch. 8, A & S)*.

(Ch. 8, A & S)

a	**True**	The low blood/gas partition coefficient of nitrous oxide (0.47) allows rapid equilibration between inspired and alveolar concentrations.
b	**False**	These contaminants of the production of nitrous oxide are removed by scrubbing at the manufacturing stage. Serious complications may result if these contaminants remain.
c	**True**	This is due to methionine synthetase depression.
d	**False**	This is not a feature of nitrous oxide usage.
e	**False**	The MAC (minimum alveolar concentration (for anaesthesia) of an agent is determined with reference to its administration in oxygen alone, and remains constant with concurrently administered agents. However, MAC values are additive.

(Ch. 22, A & S)

a	**False**	Anticholinergic agents are contraindicated in an MHS patient.
b	**True**	Vecuronium is deemed to be free of triggering potential.
c	**False**	Nitrous oxide may be employed in the MHS patient.
d	**True**	Dantrolene (up to 10 mg/kg) is the specific treatment for MH. It may also be administered preoperatively as prophylaxis in the MHS patient.
e	**True**	TIVA using propofol is one recommended technique.

66 Severe pulmonary barotrauma may be avoided by

a   a compliant reservoir bag.

b   supplying gas by pipeline rather than by cylinder.

c   use of non-interchangeable breathing system connections.

d   use of a blow-off valve set at 33 kPa in the inspiratory limb.

e   a blow-off valve set at 7 kPa on the machine.

67 The following would be noticed within 10 min of intubation of the right main bronchus:

a   high ventilation pressure.
b   increased requirement for anaesthetic vapour.

c   collapse of right upper lobe.

d   hypercapnia.

e   hypotension.

68 Ruptured pulmonary alveolus may cause

a   subcutaneous emphysema.

b   pneumopericardium.

c   superior vena cava syndrome.

d   pneumomediastinum.

e   tension pneumothorax.

(Ch. 16, A & S)

a **True** A compliant reservoir bag in the breathing circuit limits the pressure in the breathing system to approximately 30 cmH$_2$0 (3 kPa).

b **False** The pipeline pressure of 400 kPa is capable of causing severe pulmonary barotrauma.

c **False** Breathing system leaks under conditions of high pressure are more likely with interchangeable connections.

d **False** A blow-off valve at 33 kPa (which is usually incorporated into the anaesthetic machine) protects only the machine components, not the patient.

e **True** Limiting the circuit pressure to 70 cmH$_2$0 (7 kPa) with a blow-off valve obviates serious barotrauma in most patients, although it may still occur in neonates, infants and patients with some pulmonary diseases (e.g. lung bullae).

(Ch. 22, A & S)

a **True** Tidal volume for two lungs is delivered to one lung only.

b **True** During the induction phase, shunting of blood through the non-ventilated lung results in a decreased arterial anaesthetic concentration *(Ch. 7, A & S)*.

c **False** The cuff may occlude the right upper lobe bronchus, but if so, collapse supervenes at a later time.

d **False** Carbon dioxide elimination remains unchanged. Alveolar ventilation is increased slightly because dead space is reduced, but CO$_2$ elimination is impaired slightly by increased shunt; the net effect is no change during spontaneous or mechanical ventilation.

e **False** Hypotension would not be expected.

---

a **True** If a large amount of air escapes rapidly into the mediastinum, it may track into the soft tissues of the neck to produce subcutaneous emphysema.

b **False** The pericardial sac is isolated from any mediastinal air emanating from a ruptured alveolus.

c **False** Superior vena cava syndrome results from distension of the veins draining into the superior vena cava. It is associated usually with advanced carcinoma of the lungs and can be very unpleasant. It is not usually associated with pulmonary alveolar rupture.

d **True** Air escaping from ruptured alveoli may track into the mediastinum.

e **True** Tension pneumothorax is not common with a ruptured alveolus but is possible. The risk is increased in the presence of positive pressure ventilation *(Ch. 22, A & S)*.

69 Regurgitation of gastric contents is likely

a   in a patient with a hiatus hernia.

b   when the lower oesophageal barrier pressure is increased.

c   in the presence of anticholinergic drugs.
d   if the patient has not eaten solid food for 4 h.

e   in a patient following minor trauma.

70 Epidural anaesthesia

a   may be performed at any vertebral level.

b   expands the capacity of the intravascular compartment.
c   eliminates the risk of vomiting and regurgitation.

d   is associated with urinary retention.

e   may be performed using bupivacaine 0.75%.

71 After suxamethonium 50 mg, apnoea persists after 1 h:

a   probably an atypical cholinesterase is present.

b   treatment with stored blood is indicated.

c   treatment with cholinesterases is indicated.
d   this may be due to low serum K^+ concentration.

e   screening of the patient's family is mandatory.

72 In a patient with hypokalaemia

a   muscle weakness may be present.

b   the ECG shows tall T waves.
c   alkalosis exacerbates the hypokalaemia.

d   the maximum rate of replacement should not exceed 0.5 mmol/kg per hour.
e   digoxin therapy should be withdrawn.

(Ch. 31, A & S)

a **True** Loss of the anatomical sphincter action of the diaphragm increases the likelihood of regurgitation. Antacid prophylaxis is required for elective as well as emergency surgery.

b **False** Increased lower oesophageal sphincter (LOS) barrier pressure reduces the risk of reflux of gastric contents into the oesophagus.

c **True** Anticholinergic drugs reduce LOS pressure.

d **False** Under normal circumstances, gastric emptying removes solid food after 4–6 h. However, trauma occurring soon after a meal may inhibit gastric emptying for a considerable time.

e **True** Particularly when trauma occurs soon after a meal.

(Ch. 25, A & S)

a **True** However, it is performed usually in the thoracic, lumbar or caudal regions.

b **True** This is due to sympathetic blockade.

c **False** Vomiting and regurgitation are possible during epidural anaesthesia for surgery. Appropriate precautions, such as starvation and the use of antacids, should be taken.

d **True** The lack of sensory and motor function can lead to urinary retention.

e **True** Bupivacaine 0.75% is a suitable agent for epidural anaesthesia, but its use is not approved for obstetric procedures.

(Ch. 11, A & S)

a **True** A normal dose of suxamethonium produces prolonged paralysis in patients with atypical cholinesterase.

b **False** Stored blood does not contain normal plasma cholinesterase enzyme activity.

c **False** No such preparation exists.

d **False** Hypokalaemia exerts no effect upon depolarizing block. In contrast, hypokalaemia may hinder the reversibility of non-depolarizing muscle relaxants.

e **False** However, it is advisable to investigate the patient's family as well as the patient for abnormal cholinesterase variants.

(Ch. 21, A & S)

a **True** Muscle weakness and paralytic ileus may occur when total body potassium is depleted.

b **False** Tall T waves are characteristic of hyperkalaemia.

c **True** Alkalosis causes shift of extracellular potassium to the intracellular compartment and exacerbates hypokalaemia.

d **True** This permits equilibration with the intracellular compartment.

e **False** But hypokalaemia increases the risk of digoxin toxicity and calls for careful monitoring.

73 **Entrainment ratio of a Venturi oxygen mask is affected by**
a   back pressure.

b   increase in oxygen flow.

c   size of orifice.

d   peak inspiratory flow rate (PIFR).

e   dead space of the mask.

---

74 **Concerning Rotameters on a standard anaesthetic machine in the UK:**
a   oxygen is on the right when viewed from the front.

b   there is an antistatic coating on the inside of the glass tube.

c   they are less accurate if the bobbins are not rotating.
d   they employ a variable-orifice principle.

e   they are not affected by back pressure.

---

75 **Passive scavenging systems**
a   require the incorporation of a suction device.

b   can produce a negative pressure under some circumstances.

c   require the use of activated charcoal.

d   produce resistance to expiration of 2 cmH_2O at a flow rate of 30 l/min.
e   are inefficient for scavenging vapours.

(Chs. 15 and 23, A & S)

a **True** Back pressure reduces air entrainment and increases the delivered concentration of oxygen.
b **False** The entrainment ratio remains constant over a range of gas flows.
c **True** The various oxygen concentrations required are attained by using orifices of different diameter.
d **False** The PIFR does not affect the entrainment ratio. However, the total gas flow into the mask must exceed PIFR to avoid dilution of the oxygen/air mixture by air entrained through the vents in the mask.
e **False** High dead space may increase the risk of rebreathing alveolar gas when variable-performance devices are employed.

(Chs. 15 and 16, A & S)

a **False** In the flowmeter bank, oxygen is conventionally on the extreme left. However, for reasons of safety, the oxygen is added downstream from the other gases in modern anaesthetic machines.
b **True** This is to prevent sticking of the bobbin flowmeter, which would lead to inaccurate flow readings.
c **True** See **b** above.
d **True** The glass tube is tapered, and the size of the aperture increases with increasing flow; the weight of the bobbin is matched by the force caused by the pressure difference, to maintain flow.
e **False** Back pressure causes the Rotameter to under-read.

(Ch. 16, A & S)

a **False** The passive scavenging system merely vents expired gases to the outside.
b **True** Air movement at the external terminal may create negative pressure. A relief valve at −50 Pa limits this.
c **False** Activated charcoal is not part of a passive scavenging system. This adsorbs volatile agents.
d **False** The resistance to gas flow should not exceed 0.5 cmH$_2$O at 30 l/min.
e **False** Gases and volatile agents may be scavenged by such a system.

76 There is an increased risk of cardiovascular complications associated with elective surgery

a   in a patient who has had a myocardial infarction in the previous 6 months.

b   when the diastolic arterial pressure exceeds 110 mmHg in an untreated patient.

c   in patients over 70 years of age.

d   with mitral stenosis.

e   when the Goldman score exceeds 13 points.

---

77 In day-case anaesthesia

a   only patients of ASA grade I are accepted.

b   anticholinergic premedication is unnecessary.

c   thiopentone is a suitable induction agent.

d   tracheal intubation in children is hazardous.

e   local anaesthetic nerve blockade is contraindicated, because of long-lasting paralysis.

---

78 Oxygen for medical use

a   is produced by the fractional distillation of liquid air.

b   has a critical temperature of 36.5°C.

c   causes bone marrow depression with prolonged exposure.

d   is supplied in cylinders at a pressure of 137 kPa.

e   dissolves in plasma at a Pa_{O_2} of 13.3 kPa.

---

79 Complications of supraclavicular brachial plexus block include

a   pleural puncture.

b   phrenic nerve block.

c   intrathecal injection.

d   intra-arterial injection.

e   ptosis.

a **True** The risk of perioperative myocardial infarction is approximately 3–8%.
b **True** Elective surgery should be deferred in order to instigate treatment.
c **True** This increases the Goldman score.
d **False** Aortic valve stenosis, but not mitral valve stenosis, is associated with an increased risk.
e **True** The rate of major cardiac complications is between 3% and 30%.

a **False** Patients of ASA grades I and II and, occasionally, III are acceptable.
b **True**
c **False** Propofol most nearly meets the criteria of an ideal induction agent for day cases. Thiopentone would rarely be more appropriate.
d **False** Provided the correct size of tube is used, this is not hazardous.
e **False** Local analgesic techniques, with or without general anaesthesia, are useful for day-case surgery.

a **True** Commercial manufacture involves fractional distillation of liquid air.
b **False** The critical temperature of oxygen is −118°C.
c **False** Bone marrow depression is attributed to nitrous oxide. Oxygen with prolonged exposure may cause pulmonary toxicity.
d **False** The pressure in an oxygen cylinder is 13.7 MPa (137 bar; 1987 lb/in^2).
e **True** At normal arterial tension (13.3 kPa), oxygen dissolves in plasma – approximately 0.3 ml/100 ml blood.

a **True** The incidence of pneumothorax is between 0.5% and 6%.
b **True** For this reason, and the possibility of pneumothorax, bilateral supraclavicular blocks should not be undertaken.
c **False** This complication is likely only if the interscalene route is used.
d **True** The subclavian artery lies in the field of injection.
e **True** This is a manifestation of sympathetic blockade and Horner's syndrome.

80 **Fits during or after anaesthesia may be associated with**
a enflurane.
b methohexitone.

c propofol.

d ketamine.

e suxamethonium.

---

81 **Characteristics of non-depolarizing neuromuscular block include**
a post-tetanic facilitation.

b always prolonged by acidosis.

c postoperative muscle pains.

d reversible with edrophonium.

e development of dual block.

---

82 **The following are true of a Bier's block in a 60-year-old patient:**
a 30 ml lignocaine 1.5% is an acceptable dose.
b Prilocaine is not a suitable agent.
c Systemic toxicity does not occur with an effective tourniquet.

d The tourniquet can be released safely after 10 min.

e Injection in the antecubital fossa is preferred.

---

83 **Stages of anaesthesia as described by Guedel**
a refer to unpremedicated patients.
b refer to patients breathing ether.
c are divided into four planes.
d include a third stage which is divided into four planes.
e include measurement of arterial pressure and heart rate.

(Chs. 8 and 9, A & S)

a **True** Particularly with the use of concentrations greater than 3%.
b **False** Tonic excitatory movements may be associated with the use of methohexitone on induction, but fitting has not been reported.
c **True** Although propofol produces CNS depression – including reducing the duration of ECT-induced fits – there have been reports of fits after its usage. Caution is recommended with epileptic patients.
d **False** Ketamine increases intracranial pressure and cerebral metabolic rate, but has not been reported to cause fits.
e **False** Suxamethonium is a depolarizing muscle relaxant which is employed during electroconvulsive therapy to modify the external manifestations of a fit.

(Ch. 11, A & S)

a **True** Post-tetanic potentiation is a characteristic of non-depolarizing (competitive) block.
b **False** Although the action of some non-depolarizing muscle relaxants is potentiated by acidosis, the breakdown of atracurium (for example) is enhanced in the presence of acidosis.
c **False** Postoperative myalgia is associated with the use of suxamethonium.
d **True** Doses of 0.5–1 mg/kg are used for the reversal of neuromuscular blockade.
e **False** Dual blockade is associated with prolonged use of large doses of depolarizing neuromuscular blocking drugs.

(Ch. 25, A & S)

a **False** 30 ml of lignocaine 1.5% is 450 mg. This exceeds the toxic dose.
b **False** Prilocaine is the agent of choice for a Bier's block.
c **False** The leakage of local anaesthetic agent past an effective tourniquet is a well-recognized complication, and systemic toxicity can ensue.
d **False** It is recommended that the tourniquet be left in place for 20 min or longer.
e **False** High intravascular pressures can be generated, producing leakage beneath the tourniquet.

(Ch. 19, A & S)

a **False** Premedication with morphine and atropine was used.
b **True** It was described in patients breathing ether and air.
c **False** There are four stages. The third stage is divided into four planes.
d **True** See **c** above.
e **False** Guedel described the stages of anaesthesia for clinical practice alone.

84 **Injection of thiopentone and suxamethonium is followed by muscle stiffness within 15 s. This may be due to**

a atypical cholinesterase.

b myotonia congenita.

c familial periodic paralysis.

d malignant hyperpyrexia.
e dystrophia myotonica.

85 **In outpatient dental anaesthesia**

a inhalational induction with high (> 80%) concentrations of nitrous oxide is a useful method.
b a gauze throat pack should be used to obstruct oral breathing.

c focal extrasystoles are common.

d intravenous induction of anaesthesia may be undertaken with the patient seated in the dental chair.
e relative analgesia is useful because the patient need not be accompanied home.

86 **During rapid-sequence induction of anaesthesia**

a the patient must be on a tipping trolley or table.

b suction must be immediately available.
c 100% oxygen is breathed for at least 7 min before induction.

d the cricoid cartilage should be compressed.
e thiopentone is given at a rate of 1 ml/3 s.

87 **The following modify anaesthetic technique for ECT:**

a lithium treatment.
b treatment with monoamine oxidase inhibitors (MAOIs).

c cerebrovascular accident (CVA) within 3 months.
d sensitivity to propofol.

e the use of unilateral ECT.

a **False** Atypical cholinesterase prolongs the action of suxamethonium *(Ch. 11, A & S)*.
b **True** Myotonia congenita is one contraindication to administration of suxamethonium *(Ch. 40, A & S)*.
c **False** Muscle stiffness is not a characteristic of this condition *(Ch. 22, A & S)*.
d **False** Onset of muscle stiffness would be later than 15 s.
e **True** This is another contraindication.

(Ch. 34, A & S)

a **False** This outdated technique has no place in modern practice. The F_{O_2} must be at least 0.3.
b **True** Correct placement is essential to obstruct oral breathing whilst maintaining a clear nasopharyngeal passage.
c **True** Arrhythmias occur in approximately 30% of patients and are usually unifocal extrasystoles.
d **False** Intravenous induction should be undertaken only in the supine patient. There is a risk of hypotension in the seated position.
e **True** Relative analgesia employs a concentration of approximately 30% N_2O and recovery is rapid. Verbal contact with the patient is maintained throughout.

(Ch. 31, A & S)

a **True** It is essential to be able to initiate a head-down tilt and employ pharyngeal suction to assist gravity drainage of any regurgitated gastric contents away from the laryngeal inlet.
b **True** See **a** above.
c **False** Preoxygenation should be employed for 3–5 min. Four maximal (vital capacity) breaths are an acceptable alternative.
d **True** Cricoid pressure should be applied by a competent assistant.
e **False** Rapid-sequence induction employs the use of a predetermined dose of induction agent injected rapidly.

(Ch. 29, A & S)

a **True** Lithium potentiates the action of neuromuscular blocking drugs.
b **False** Opioids (and particularly pethidine) which interact with MAOIs are not used routinely in anaesthesia for ECT.
c **True** CVA within 3 months is a contraindication to the use of ECT.
d **False** Propofol is probably not indicated for induction of anaesthesia for ECT as there is some evidence that it modifies the convulsion.
e **False** The technique of anaesthesia for unilateral ECT is no different from that for bilateral ECT.

88 Entonox

a is stored in cylinders at 13.7 MPa.

b is approved for use by unsupervised midwives by the UKCC (United Kingdom Central Council for Nursing, Midwifery and Health Visiting).

c should be stored below −8°C.

d may depress bone marrow following prolonged administration.

e should not be used in the presence of a closed cavity pneumothorax.

89 Postoperative hypoxaemia may occur as a result of

a mild hypercapnia.

b nitrous oxide diffusion.

c central depression of ventilation.

d increased $\dot{V}/\dot{Q}$ mismatch.

e fentanyl given 2 h previously.

90 Bupivacaine

a causes depolarization of nerve membranes.

b is contraindicated for IVRA.

c has a longer duration of action than lignocaine.

d is metabolized in the liver.

e is unsuitable for intrathecal use.

(Ch. 15, A & S)

a **True** The normal filling pressure of a cylinder of air, oxygen, and premixed nitrous oxide and oxygen (Entonox) is 13.7 MPa (approximately 2000 lb/in^2).

b **True** It is used widely in delivery suites *(Ch. 32, A & S)*.

c **False** If Entonox is stored below $-7°C$, it may separate into its constituent parts. This is the pseudo-critical temperature.

d **True** The nitrous oxide component of Entonox is responsible for the bone marrow depression following prolonged administration. This is unlikely in obstetric practice.

e **True** Nitrous oxide is contraindicated in the presence of air in a closed cavity such as a pneumothorax.

(Ch. 23, A & S)

a **False** The influence of mild hypercapnia on oxygen transport is minimal.

b **False** One would not expect diffusion hypoxia to last more than 10 min.

c **True** Due to the persistent action of volatile anaesthetic agents, opioid analgesics, benzodiazepines, barbiturates, etc.

d **True** Anaesthesia leads to $\dot{V}/\dot{Q}$ imbalance, which persists into the postoperative period. The effect on Pa_{O_2} is exacerbated by a decrease in cardiac output and hypoventilation.

e **True** If given in high doses, fentanyl may produce depression of ventilation at this time.

(Ch. 14, A & S)

a **False** Local anaesthetic agents prevent depolarization of the nerve membranes, probably by blocking the sodium–potassium channels.

b **True** Bupivacaine is contraindicated for IVRA. Fatalities have been reported following cuff failure.

c **True** It has a relative duration two to four times that of lignocaine.

d **True** It is an amide-linked agent and is metabolized by amidases in the liver.

e **False** It is suitable for intrathecal use, in either plain or hyperbaric formulation.

91 **The neuromuscular blocking drugs in clinical use**
a are all metabolized by acetylcholine.
b exhibit tetanic fade if the block is depolarizing.

c produce phase II block when curare-like drugs are used.

d produce post-tetanic facilitation with curare-like drugs.

e produce initial fasciculation when the drug is an agonist.

92 **After massive inhalation of gastric acid the following may result:**
a lung abscess.

b type I respiratory failure.

c bacteraemia.

d hypovolaemia.

e destruction of surfactant.

93 **Boyle's law**
a relates pressure to temperature.
b applies only to ideal gases.

c concerns a given mass of gas.
d relates pressure to volume.
e refers to a given volume of gas.

94 **Critical pressure is**
a the pressure above which a liquid cannot evaporate.

b the pressure above which a cylinder must not be filled.

c the pressure of vapour in equilibrium with liquid at critical temperature.

d the pressure below which Entonox must not be stored.

e approximately 50 atm for oxygen.

(Ch. 11, A & S)

a **False** Acetylcholine is the normal transmitter of neuromuscular signals.
b **False** A tetanic fade is associated with non-depolarizing neuromuscular blocking drugs.
c **False** Phase II block occurs with repeated doses of depolarizing agents, not curare-like drugs.
d **True** This is a characteristic feature of non-depolarizing blocking drugs.
e **True** Fasciculation is a characteristic of depolarizing neuromuscular blocking drugs which mimic the action of acetylcholine.

(Ch. 4, D; Chs. 22 and 31, A & S)

a **True** Lung abscesses may form if death does not precede their development.
b **False** Initially, type II respiratory failure (with high Pa_{CO_2} and low Pa_{O_2}) may develop – possibly followed by type I.
c **True** Pulmonary complications arise initially from a chemical pneumonitis, but bacteraemia may supervene.
d **True** Hypovolaemia occurs secondary to extracellular fluid loss into the lung tissue.
e **True** This leads to the adult respiratory distress syndrome *(Ch. 41, A & S)*.

(Ch. 15, A & S)

a **False** Boyle's law applies at constant temperature.
b **True** Gases which are well above their critical temperature behave usually as ideal gases.
c **True** It relates to a fixed mass of gas.
d **True** $P \times V = k$ is the equation for Boyle's law.
e **False** It does not refer to a fixed volume of gas.

(Ch. 15, A & S)

a **False** The critical pressure is that pressure required to liquefy a gas at its critical temperature.
b **False** A cylinder is frequently filled with gas to a pressure above its critical pressure, e.g. an oxygen cylinder.
c **True** When a liquid is at its critical temperature, it exists in equilibrium as liquid and vapour. The critical pressure is the pressure above the liquid at its critical temperature.
d **False** Entonox should not be stored below what is termed the pseudo-critical temperature.
e **True** The critical temperature of oxygen is approximately –118°C, and the critical pressure is approximately 50 atm (5 MPa).

95 **Junctional rhythm accompanied by bradycardia**

   a requires immediate treatment and is dangerous.

   b occurs commonly during anaesthesia with halothane.

   c can be produced by hypoxaemia.

   d can be produced by light anaesthesia.

   e may be responsive to atropine.

96 **Humidification of inspired gases reduces**

   a drying and crusting of bronchial secretions.

   b respiratory heat loss.

   c respiratory water loss.

   d anatomical dead space.

   e likelihood of infection.

97 **During external chest compression in cardiopulmonary resuscitation (CPR)**

   a the heel of the hand should be over the cardiac apex.

   b the fingers should be in close contact with the chest wall.

   c the elbows should be flexed.

   d lung inflation should be performed every 15 compressions.

   e a full sequence of basic life support (BLS) should be completed before considering defibrillation.

98 **Antagonism of neuromuscular block**

   a can be achieved with edrophonium.

   b is unnecessary if the train-of-four (TOF) ratio is < 0.3.

   c occurs only if atropine is used with neostigmine.

   d is unnecessary if the patient can sustain a head-lift for 5 s.

   e can be achieved with physostigmine.

(Ch. 22, A & S)

a **False** Provided that the arterial pressure is maintained, there is no need for immediate treatment – but close monitoring is essential.
b **True** Junctional rhythm is common during halothane anaesthesia.
c **False** Hypoxaemia usually produces tachycardia in the early stages.
d **False** Light anaesthesia is usually accompanied by tachycardia.
e **True** Atropine increases the rate of depolarization of the sinoatrial node, because of vagal inhibition.

(Chs. 15 and 33, A & S)

a **True** Dry crusts may be a problem after prolonged inhalation of dry gases.
b **True** Heat loss is reduced by humidification.
c **True** The loss of respiratory water (necessary to humidify dry gases) is reduced when inhaled gases are humidified.
d **False** Humidification has no effect on dead space.
e **False** The likelihood of infection may be increased if humidifiers are sterilized inadequately. Disposable pre-sterilized heat and moisture exchangers for single patient use are commonly employed to obviate this.

(Ch. 43, A & S)

a **False** The heel of the hand should be placed on the lower third of the sternum.
b **False** The fingers should be raised so as not to injure the ribs.
c **False** The elbows should be locked in extension to reduce fatigue.
d **True** When there is only one resuscitator, two expired-air lung inflations should be performed after every 15 chest compressions.
e **False** Early defibrillation is important. In the operating theatre or ICU (for example) defibrillation may be used prior to BLS if a defibrillator is to hand.

(Ch. 11, A & S)

a **True** Edrophonium is a short-acting anticholinesterase.
b **False** TOF ratio should be greater than 0.7 to achieve adequate neuromuscular transmission.
c **False** Atropine is used to counteract the unwanted muscarinic actions of anticholinesterases.
d **True** Sustained head-lift is a useful clinical indication of adequate neuromuscular function.
e **False** Physostigmine is an anticholinesterase with central actions, and is unsuitable for reversal of neuromuscular block.

99 **Concerning muscle relaxants:**
a atracurium is broken down largely by plasma cholinesterase.

b vecuronium is a steroid.

c atracurium causes less histamine release than vecuronium.
d mivacurium is broken down largely by plasma cholinesterase.

e rocuronium can be used safely in patients with impaired renal function.

---

100 **Success of cricoid pressure in prevention of regurgitation of gastric contents depends upon**
a absence of a nasogastric tube.

b an intact cricoid cartilage.

c the oesophagus being pressed against the vertebral body.

d preoperative administration of H_2-antagonists.

e preoxygenation for 5 min.

(Ch. 11, A & S)

a **False** Atracurium is broken down by Hofmann degradation, which is pH-and temperature-dependent. A small amount undergoes ester hydrolysis.

b **True** But it possesses none of the steroid actions associated with adrenocortical steroids.

c **False** Atracurium, alcuronium and tubocurarine may release histamine.

d **True** In patients with atypical cholinesterase, prolongation of action is seen.

e **False** In common with pancuronium, rocuronium is excreted renally. It is unsuitable for use in renally impaired patients.

(Ch. 31, A & S)

a **True** A nasogastric tube renders the lower oesophageal sphincter incompetent, and may prevent efficient occlusion of the oesophagus behind the cricoid cartilage.

b **True** In contrast to other tracheal rings, the cricoid cartilage encircles the trachea and permits oesophageal compression.

c **True** The oesophagus is compressed between the cricoid cartilage and the body of the sixth cervical vertebra.

d **False** H_2-antagonists increase the pH of gastric contents, but do not influence the risk of regurgitation.

e **False** This is an important precaution before rapid-sequence induction, but does not influence the efficacy of cricoid pressure.

5. Examination 1

1 **The following signs may be present in chronic obstructive airways disease (COAD):**
   a diminished area of cardiac dullness.

   b palpable liver edge.
   c finger clubbing.

   d cyanosis.

   e increased inspiratory, rather than expiratory, effort.

---

2 **In respect of a cylinder of anaesthetic gas:**
   a The pressure inside a full nitrous oxide cylinder is 120 atm.
   b The pressure is reduced to a pipeline value of 60 lb/in^2.

   c The filling ratio of a nitrous oxide cylinder is the ratio of weight of nitrous oxide to the weight of water it would hold.
   d Helium cylinders are bright orange in colour.
   e Entonox should be stored at a temperature above –7°C.

---

3 **Impurities of nitrous oxide produced during manufacture include**
   a ammonia.

   b chlorine.
   c nitric oxide.
   d nitrogen dioxide.

   e nitrogen.

(Ch. 4, D)

a	**True**	A diminished area of cardiac dullness is a feature of emphysema, which may occur in COAD.
b	**True**	Cor pulmonale is a late feature of COAD.
c	**False**	Finger clubbing may occur in the presence of carcinoma, chronic intrathoracic suppuration, fibrosing alveolitis and a number of other conditions, but not in COAD.
d	**True**	This may occur in severe COAD. There may be associated polycythaemia.
e	**False**	Air trapping is a feature of COAD. This occurs in the expiratory phase, with increased respiratory effort.

(Chs. 15 and 16, A & S)

a	**False**	The pressure is 44 bar (4.5 MPa).
b	**True**	400 kPa (60 lb/in^2) is the pressure which is applied to the needle valves of the Rotameters.
c	**True**	The filling ratio is normally about 67%.
d	**False**	Helium cylinders are brown.
e	**True**	Separation of liquid nitrous oxide occurs below this temperature, the pseudo-critical temperature for Entonox.

(Ch. 8, A & S)

a	**True**	Nitrous oxide is produced by heating ammonium nitrate. Ammonia is a potential impurity.
b	**False**	There is no chlorine or chloride involved in the reaction.
c	**True**	Nitric oxide (NO) is a higher oxide of nitrogen.
d	**True**	Nitrogen dioxide (NO_2) is a higher oxide of nitrogen. The higher oxides dissolve in water, form nitrous and nitric acids, and are toxic.
e	**True**	

4 **In diabetes mellitus**
  a insulin requirements increase during pregnancy.
  b postural hypotension may occur.
  c corneal opacities occur.
  d microvascular complications occur, but only in the elderly.

  e metformin treatment may lead to acidosis.

5 **Nitrous oxide**
  a is stored as a liquid.

  b has a molecular weight of 44.
  c is manufactured by heating ammonium nitrate.

  d supports combustion.

  e may contain contaminants which may be detected by starch-iodide paper.

6 **Treatment of hypokalaemia is necessary**
  a after cardiac bypass surgery.

  b during treatment for diabetic ketoacidosis.

  c after major burns.

  d after depolarizing relaxants.

  e during carbenoxolone therapy.

7 **In acute appendicitis**
  a there is usually obstruction of the appendix lumen.
  b the pain starts typically in the right iliac fossa.

  c the pain is aggravated by movement.
  d nausea or vomiting is usually present.

  e the white blood cell count may be normal.

(Ch. 8, D)

a	**True**	Blood sugar concentration may be labile during pregnancy.
b	**True**	This is a result of autonomic neuropathy.
c	**False**	There is no increased incidence of cataract in diabetics.
d	**False**	Microangiopathy is independent of age (and possibly independent of diabetic control).
e	**True**	Lactic acidosis is a recognized complication of treatment with biguanides, of which metformin is the only one available in the UK.

(Ch. 8, A & S)

a	**True**	It has a critical temperature of 36.4°C and is stored usually as a liquid at a pressure of approximately 4.5 MPa.
b	**True**	
c	**True**	The decomposition of ammonium nitrate leads to the formation of nitrous oxide plus water.
d	**True**	Whilst not itself flammable, nitrous oxide supports combustion.
e	**True**	Starch-iodide paper turns blue in the presence of the contaminants of nitrous oxide manufacture.

---

a	**True**	This is common after cardiac bypass surgery, and potassium supplementation is usually required *(Ch. 39, A & S)*.
b	**True**	Insulin administration activates sodium–potassium exchange in the distal tubule of the kidney, resulting in hypokalaemia *(Ch. 40, A & S)*.
c	**False**	Hyperkalaemia would be expected as a result of massive cell destruction. The use of suxamethonium is contraindicated *(Ch. 35, A & S)*.
d	**False**	Suxamethonium, the only available depolarizing relaxant in the UK, causes mild transient hyperkalaemia.
e	**True**	Carbenoxolone has aldosterone-like effects *(Ch. 5, D)*.

(Ch. 9, D)

a	**True**	This is caused by swelling of lymphoid tissue in the walls.
b	**False**	Initially the pain is central and moves later to the right iliac fossa.
c	**True**	Particularly with peritoneal inflammation.
d	**True**	But vomiting is less severe than that associated with intestinal obstruction.
e	**False**	Fever and toxicity are associated with an elevated white cell count.

8 **The following factors favour rapid induction with an inhalational agent:**
a   high blood/gas partition coefficient.

b   low alveolar ventilation.
c   low SVP at 20°C.

d   high concentrations of catecholamines.

e   the second gas effect.

9 **Atrial flutter**
a   is caused most commonly by ischaemic heart disease.

b   is identified by 'f' waves at 20/s.
c   is characterized by a regular arterial pulse.

d   must not be treated by DC cardioversion.
e   may be prevented by prophylactic administration of digoxin.

10 **Malignant hyperthermia (MH) has the following features:**
a   muscle rigidity.

b   hyperkalaemia.
c   relaxation following alcuronium.
d   increased base excess.
e   family history.

11 **The following drugs are halogenated ethers:**
a   isoflurane.
b   diethyl ether.
c   enflurane.
d   halothane.
e   seroflurane.

(Ch. 7, A & S)

a	**False**	A low blood/gas partition coefficient (e.g. nitrous oxide) is necessary for rapid induction with an inhalational agent.
b	**False**	Increasing alveolar ventilation increases the rate of induction.
c	**False**	The saturated vapour pressure at 20°C indicates the maximum concentration of agent that may be administered to a patient. This may limit the use of 'over pressure' to increase the speed of induction.
d	**False**	These increase cardiac output and therefore decrease the rate of induction.
e	**True**	Rapid uptake of a second gas (nitrous oxide) from the alveoli allows the alveolar concentration of a volatile agent to increase more rapidly in the presence of a high concentration of nitrous oxide, thus favouring rapid induction of anaesthesia *(Ch. 8, A & S)*.

(Ch. 3, D)

a	**False**	Mitral valve disease is the commonest cause in younger patients. In the elderly, there may be no apparent cause or it may occur secondary to hypertension or ischaemic heart disease.
b	**False**	The atrial rate is usually about 300/min.
c	**True**	There is usually a regular atrioventricular (AV) block but the ratio may vary between 2:1 and 4:1.
d	**False**	Low energy cardioversion may be effective.
e	**True**	

(Ch. 22, A & S)

a	**True**	Increased muscle tone may occur following suxamethonium, particularly in young patients.
b	**True**	Hyperkalaemia results from cellular breakdown.
c	**False**	Muscle relaxants have no effect on muscle itself.
d	**False**	Acidosis occurs.
e	**True**	Susceptibility to MH is inherited as an autosomal dominant with variable penetrance.

(Ch. 8, A & S)

a	**True**	Isoflurane is 1-chloro-2,2,2-trifluoroethyl difluoromethyl ether.
b	**False**	It is unsubstituted.
c	**True**	Enflurane is an isomer of isoflurane.
d	**False**	Halothane is a halogenated ethane.
e	**True**	It is a substituted methylpropylether.

12   The following are true of anaesthesia in a patient chronically on dialysis:
a Suxamethonium is contraindicated.

b Halothane may cause dose-related tubular damage.
c Anaesthesia should be postponed if the haemoglobin concentration is <10 g/dl.
d Antihypertensive treatment should be continued preoperatively.
e A sterile laryngoscope should be used.

13   Pulsation in the neck is probably venous if it
a is diffuse.
b increases with abdominal pressure.
c is readily palpable.
d varies with ventilation.
e varies with posture.

14   Naloxone may completely antagonize respiratory depression produced by
a levorphanol.

b doxapram.
c pentazocine.

d nalbuphine.

e buprenorphine.

15   The following MAC values are correct at normal atmospheric pressure:
a nitrous oxide – 105%.
b halothane – 1.2%.
c enflurane – 1.7%.
d isoflurane – 1.7%.
e sevoflurane – 1.0%.

(Ch. 40, A & S)

a **False** Provided that serum potassium concentration is normal, there is no contraindication.
b **False** Halothane is not nephrotoxic.
c **False** A haemoglobin concentration of less than 10 g/dl is commonly encountered in patients with chronic renal failure.
d **True**
e **False** The oropharynx is not sterile.

(Ch. 3, D)

a **True** This is observed best with the patient reclining at an angle of 45°.
b **True** This is the hepatojugular reflux.
c **False** Venous pressure is impalpable.
d **True** Intrathoracic pressure is transmitted to the intrathoracic veins.
e **True** When pulsation is very high in cardiac failure, it may be apparent only when the patient stands.

(Ch. 10, A & S)

a **True** This is an opioid agonist and its action is antagonized by naloxone. It has a prolonged duration of action (6–10 h), whilst that of naloxone is 15–20 min – therefore a naloxone infusion may be required.
b **False** Doxapram is an analeptic respiratory stimulant.
c **True** Naloxone reverses respiratory depression produced by pentazocine, which is a μ-antagonist and a κ-agonist.
d **True** Nalbuphine is a partial agonist at κ-receptors and an antagonist at μ-receptors. Its actions are antagonized by naloxone, which is an antagonist at μ-, κ- and δ-receptors.
e **False** Buprenorphine is a partial agonist at μ-receptors and is therefore antagonized theoretically by naloxone. However, buprenorphine has an extremely high receptor affinity and in standard dosage naloxone is relatively ineffective.

(Appendix. II A & S)

a **True**
b **False** Halothane – 0.75%.
c **True**
d **False** Isoflurane – 1.15%.
e **False** Sevoflurane – 2.0%.

16   The pressure gauge on a nitrous oxide cylinder

   a   may be calibrated in bar.
   b   is essential for assessment of the quantity of residual gas in the cylinder.
   c   shows a constant pressure as gas runs steadily out of the cylinder at a flow rate of 10 l/min, provided that the cylinder still contains liquid nitrous oxide.
   d   may indicate an increase in pressure after the cylinder is turned off after continuous use.
   e   measures absolute pressure.

17   Complications of diabetes mellitus include

   a   renal papillary necrosis.

   b   abnormal response to a Valsalva manoeuvre.
   c   fat atrophy.
   d   Dupuytren's contracture.
   e   chronic pancreatitis.

18   In comparison with thiopentone, etomidate

   a   is more dangerous on intra-arterial injection.
   b   is more painful on i.v. injection.
   c   causes more cardiovascular depression.
   d   causes more abnormal muscle movements.
   e   causes more adrenal suppression.

19   Mapleson's classification of anaesthetic breathing systems

   a   describes four systems: A, B, C, D.
   b   classifies the Bain system as a Mapleson C.
   c   describes the Magill system as requiring a fresh gas flow rate equal to the minute volume during spontaneous ventilation.

   d   describes the T-piece as a Mapleson D.
   e   describes the T-piece system as requiring a fresh gas flow rate of 1.5–2 times the patient's minute volume during spontaneous ventilation.

(Ch. 15, A & S)

a **True** However, the gauge is frequently calibrated in kPa.
b **False** Only the weight of the cylinder provides an indication of the amount of residual nitrous oxide.
c **False** At high flow rates, pressure in the cylinder may decrease because of evaporation of nitrous oxide and a consequent decrease in temperature and saturated vapour pressure.
d **True** The cylinder's temperature increases to that of the ambient temperature.
e **False** The pressure gauge of a cylinder measures gauge pressure (the pressure in excess of atmospheric pressure).

(Ch. 8, D)

a **False** Glomerulosclerosis is the characteristic renal lesion complicating diabetes mellitus.
b **True** This is caused by autonomic neuropathy.
c **True** This may occur at insulin injection sites.
d **False** This is associated with alcoholic cirrhosis.
e **False** Approximately 20% of patients with chronic pancreatitis develop diabetes mellitus.

(Ch. 9, A & S)

a **False** There are fewer sequelae than after intra-arterial thiopentone.
b **True** This may be reduced by pre-injection of lignocaine.
c **False** Hypotension is less than that associated with thiopentone.
d **True** Movement, coughing and hiccuping occur more commonly.
e **True** Cortisol synthesis and response to ACTH are suppressed.

(Ch. 16, A & S)

a **False** Systems A to F are described in the Mapleson classification.
b **False** The Bain system is an example of a Mapleson D.
c **False** The Magill system functions efficiently during spontaneous ventilation, when fresh gas flow rate is equal to the alveolar minute volume.
d **False** The T-piece is an example of a Mapleson E system.
e **False** The T-piece requires a fresh gas flow rate of 2.5–3 times the patient's minute volume during spontaneous ventilation.

20 **The following statements are true of total intravenous anaesthesia:**
   a Ketamine is an appropriate agent.

   b A loading dose of anaesthetic agent is necessary to achieve smooth anaesthesia.
   c Target-controlled infusion (TCI) rates based on measured plasma concentrations may be used.
   d The patient breathes air/oxygen.
   e Propofol is a suitable agent in the elderly.

21 **The following may cause hypokalaemia:**
   a intravenous digoxin.
   b Addisonian crisis.
   c hyperventilation.

   d spironolactone therapy.

   e respiratory acidosis.

22 **Hypoalbuminaemia**
   a is associated with reduction in serum concentration of ionized calcium.
   b is a manifestation of hypopituitarism.
   c may cause tetany.
   d may be a feature of carcinoma of the oesophagus.

   e may develop in hepatic cirrhosis.

23 **4 h postoperatively, a patient breathing air is distressed, with heart rate 100 beats/min, BP 170/100 mmHg, Pa_{O_2}, 9 kPa, Pa_{CO_2} 7 kPa, HCO_3^- 28 mmol/l. This is compatible with:**
   a segmental pulmonary collapse.

   b septicaemia.

   c overtransfusion.

   d hypoventilation.
   e metabolic acidosis.

(Ch. 9, A & S)

a	**True**	Dissociative anaesthesia occurs. Premedication with atropine is recommended.
b	**True**	This is a simple pharmacokinetic principle *(Ch. 7, A & S)*.
c	**False**	TCI uses predicted plasma concentrations.
d	**True**	An increased F_{IO_2} is recommended during general anaesthesia.
e	**True**	Although a reduced dose rate is advisable.

(Ch. 21, A & S; Ch. 5, D)

a	**False**	But hypokalaemia potentiates the toxic effects of digoxin.
b	**False**	Addisonian crisis is associated with hyponatraemia *(Ch. 8, D)*.
c	**True**	Hyperventilation results in alkalosis and a shift of potassium from extracellular to intracellular fluid.
d	**False**	Spironolactone is a potassium-sparing diuretic and is an aldosterone antagonist.
e	**False**	The mechanism is the reverse of that associated with hyperventilation.

(Ch. 5, D)

a	**False**	The concentration of ionized calcium is increased because of decreased protein binding.
b	**False**	
c	**False**	Tetany is a manifestation of hypocalcaemia *(Ch. 8, D)*.
d	**True**	Patients with carcinoma of the oesophagus may be hypoalbuminaemic because of chronic undernutrition, and may benefit from preoperative parenteral feeding *(Ch. 38, A & S)*.
e	**True**	Because of impaired albumin synthesis by the liver.

(Ch. 23, A & S)

a	**False**	Carbon dioxide excretion in this condition would be relatively unaffected.
b	**False**	The arterial pressure and Pa_{CO_2} are incompatible with this diagnosis.
c	**False**	Hypercapnia is unlikely with overtransfusion, unless the patient develops gross cardiac and respiratory failure.
d	**True**	The slightly elevated bicarbonate suggests a chronic element.
e	**False**	In metabolic acidosis, the plasma bicarbonate concentration is decreased.

24 **Pulse oximetry**

a measures oxygen saturation.

b locates the isobestic point of haemoglobin.

c functions poorly on negroid skin.
d is inaccurate in the presence of carboxyhaemoglobin.

e is inaccurate in the presence of fetal haemoglobin.

25 **The plasma concentration of a drug which undergoes metabolism and elimination**

a decreases linearly with time after bolus i.v. administration.

b plotted against response gives a sigmoid curve.

c declines by 50% in proportion to the initial concentration.

d increases rapidly during constant i.v. infusion.

e at steady state with a constant infusion rate, is inversely proportional to the clearance.

26 **Pancuronium**

a does not cross the placenta in clinically significant amounts.

b causes tachycardia.
c causes less hypotension than curare.

d may cause prolonged paralysis in a patient taking streptomycin.

e causes dilation of the pupil.

(Ch. 20, A & S)

a	True	Absorption of light measured at two distinct wavelengths permits calculation of saturation.
b	False	This is the wavelength at which absorption of light is identical for oxygenated and reduced haemoglobin.
c	False	
d	True	Carboxyhaemoglobin and methaemoglobin result in inaccuracy.
e	False	

(Ch. 7, A & S)

a	False	The plot of drug concentration against time varies with the drug and its metabolic pathways. It is usually an exponential decay.
b	False	A linear plot of plasma concentration against response gives a hyperbolic curve; plot of the logarithm of concentration against response gives a sigmoid curve.
c	False	The half-life is inversely proportional to the elimination rate constant.
d	False	A constant i.v. infusion results eventually in a relatively constant plasma concentration, depending on the rate of administration and the rate of excretion of the drug. A bolus i.v. dose gives a rapid increase in plasma concentration.
e	True	Infusion rate = $C_{SS} \times Cl$ (concentration at steady state × clearance).

(Ch. 11, A & S)

a	True	Pancuronium crosses the placenta, but this is not clinically significant.
b	True	Pancuronium has significant sympathomimetic activity.
c	True	Curare may cause marked hypotension because of histamine release and ganglion blockade.
d	True	The aminoglycoside antibiotics possess neuromuscular blocking properties, and this may potentiate the action of non-depolarizing neuromuscular blocking drugs *(Ch. 18, A & S)*.
e	False	Amongst the non-depolarizing drugs, curare has the greatest ganglion-blocking action and it may cause dilation of the pupil, an effect not produced by other drugs in this class.

27 **Paroxysmal supraventricular tachycardia is**
a usually the result of organic heart disease.
b associated with the loss of P waves on the ECG.
c often terminated by carotid sinus massage.
d often terminated by treatment with verapamil.
e sometimes associated with polyuria.

28 **The following factors affect flowmeter readings (of the Rotameter type):**
a water condensation inside the tube.

b dirt on the bobbin.
c static electricity.

d gas escaping past the bobbin.

e the use of a gas different from that for which the Rotameter was calibrated.

29 **Concerning anaesthetic apparatus:**
a An oxygen-failure warning device must operate even in the absence of nitrous oxide.
b The Boyle machine can be classed as an intermittent-flow device.
c With vaporizers in series, the enflurane vaporizer should be closer to the Rotameters than the halothane vaporizer.

d When a restriction in the outflow of a Rotameter causes pressure build-up, the actual flow is greater than indicated.
e The Ruben valve is of the non-rebreathing type.

30 **The following are causes of metabolic acidosis:**
a ureterocolic fistula.
b vomiting.
c diarrhoea.

d CO_2 retention.
e metformin therapy.

(Ch. 3, D)

a	**False**	But left ventricular failure may accompany the arrhythmia.
b	**False**	Atrial depolarization is normal but accelerated.
c	**True**	This simple expedient may be the only treatment required.
d	**True**	This may be indicated if the attack is more severe.
e	**True**	This may be a feature of prolonged attacks.

(Ch. 16, A & S)

a	**True**	Water condensing inside the tube causes the bobbin to stick and results in loss of accuracy.
b	**True**	Sticking may occur as a result of debris on the bobbin.
c	**True**	Static electricity inhibits movement of the bobbin inside the tube and leads to inaccuracy. The inside of the tube is therefore coated with an antistatic film.
d	**False**	Gas escaping past the bobbin through the variable orifice is the principle underlying the operation of the flowmeter.
e	**True**	Calibration is affected by gas viscosity at low flow rates, and density at high rates. Thus a flowmeter is calibrated specifically for one gas.

(Ch. 16, A & S)

a	**True**	A safe device is that which relies upon a reservoir of compressed oxygen, which is filled from the oxygen supply.
b	**False**	A continuous flow of gases is supplied by the Boyle machine.
c	**False**	The less volatile agent should be placed downstream, to avoid contamination of the second agent. Modern machines prevent the use of two agents in series.
d	**False**	The Rotameter over-reads.
e	**True**	But non-rebreathing valves may not be 100% efficient.

(Ch. 5, D)

a	**True**	Caused by colonic absorption of hydrogen ions.
b	**False**	Vomiting results usually in metabolic alkalosis.
c	**True**	Diarrhoea leads to loss of bicarbonate ions and metabolic acidosis may result.
d	**False**	This causes respiratory acidosis.
e	**True**	Metformin is associated with lactic acidosis.

31 **In the acute phase following sudden massive haemorrhage there is**
a   a reduction in CVP.
b   widespread vasoconstriction.

c   an increase in the volume of interstitial fluid.

d   decreased secretion of antidiuretic hormone (ADH).

e   increased plasma concentration of aldosterone.

---

32 **The following drugs are peripherally acting adrenergic blockers:**
a   clonidine.
b   reserpine.

c   tolazoline.

d   droperidol.

e   methyldopa.

---

33 **Water intoxication is associated with**
a   confusion.

b   coma.
c   convulsions.
d   increased heart size.
e   hypokalaemia.

---

34 **A supraclavicular brachial plexus block**
a   can be carried out safely using 30 ml of lignocaine 2% with adrenaline 1:100 000.
b   results in cutaneous anaesthesia in the whole of the upper limb.

c   may cause Horner's syndrome.

d   has a slower onset time than an axillary block.
e   is contraindicated in haemophilia.

(Ch. 31, A & S)

a **True** The CVP is a good indicator of intravascular volume.
b **True** Vasoconstriction is part of the sympathetic response to haemorrhage.
c **False** A shift of interstitial fluid into the intravascular compartment would be expected.
d **False** There is increased ADH secretion in response to reduction in stretch receptor activity of the atrial volume receptors.
e **False** Aldosterone is secreted in response to increased plasma concentrations of angiotensin, which result from release of renin from the kidney.

(Ch. 12, A & S)

a **False** Clonidine is a peripheral and central α_2-agonist.
b **False** Reserpine acts centrally to cause depletion of neurotransmitters.
c **True** Tolazoline is a peripherally acting alpha-adrenergic blocking drug.
d **True** The butyrophenones possess mild alpha-adrenergic blocking activity.
e **False** The action of methyldopa – a false transmitter – is almost entirely central.

(Ch. 21, A & S)

a **True** This is caused by cerebral oedema, resulting from hyponatraemia.
b **True** This may result also from cerebral oedema.
c **True** These may occur in severe water intoxication.
d **False**
e **False** Hyponatraemia occurs.

(Ch. 25, A & S)

a **False** The maximum safe dose of lignocaine (200 mg; 500 mg with adrenaline) is exceeded if lignocaine 2% is used.
b **False** The intercostobrachial nerve is not included. This carries cutaneous sensation from the upper medial part of the limb.
c **True** Horner's syndrome is a frequent complication of brachial plexus block.
d **False** Axillary block is associated with a prolonged time of onset.
e **True** Regional anaesthetic techniques are contraindicated in the presence of coagulopathies.

35 **The MAC of an agent varies with**
  a   age.

  b   hypothermia.
  c   lipid-solubility of the agent.

  d   presence of nitrous oxide.

  e   premedication.

---

36 **The following changes support a diagnosis of obstructive jaundice:**
  a   increased serum acid phosphatase.
  b   increase in red cell fragility.
  c   stercobilinogen deficiency.

  d   increased urobilinogen.

  e   serum aspartate aminotransferase (AST) concentration < 100 iu/l.

---

37 **A serum sodium concentration of 127 mmol/l and a potassium concentration of 6.8 mmol/l may be found in the following conditions:**
  a   acute renal failure.
  b   Cushing's syndrome.

  c   hypopituitarism.
  d   pyloric stenosis.
  e   renal tubular acidosis.

(Ch. 8, A & S)

a **True**   The MAC of an agent increases following birth, peaks around the time of puberty and thereafter decreases slowly.
b **True**   The MAC of an agent decreases in the hypothermic patient.
c **True**   There is a linear relationship between oil/gas partition coefficient and MAC.
d **True**   Nitrous oxide reduces MAC, which is determined by reference to the inhalational agent in oxygen alone.
e **True**   Premedication reduces the requirements for an inhalational agent. MAC is determined normally in the unpremedicated state.

(Ch. 10, D)

a **False**   Serum alkaline phosphatase concentration is increased.
b **False**
c **True**   Stercobilinogen is decreased and steatorrhoea occurs in obstructive jaundice.
d **False**   Urobilinogen is conjugated bilirubin, which is reabsorbed via the gut and excreted in the urine; thus its concentration is decreased in obstructive jaundice.
e **True**   Aspartate aminotransferase is liberated following hepatocellular damage, but it may increase in severe obstructive jaundice.

(Chs. 5 and 8, D)

a **True**   Hyperkalaemia is a feature of renal failure.
b **False**   Sodium is retained as a result of increased corticosteroid secretion in Cushing's syndrome.
c **True**   Hypopituitarism is one of the causes of Addison's disease.
d **False**   Pyloric stenosis results in alkalosis and hypokalaemia.
e **False**   In renal tubular acidosis, the underlying defect is diminished sodium/hydrogen ion exchange. Potassium depletion is common in either type 1 (distal) or type 2 (proximal) renal tubular acidosis.

38 On a modern UK anaesthetic machine

a the oxygen alarm does not sound if the nitrous oxide is disconnected.

b the wall gas pipeline supply should be disconnected for the duration of the preoperative check.

c the TRITEC vaporizer cannot be used when the circle system and CO_2 absorber are in use.

d when checking for leaks with the common gas outlet blocked, the oxygen flush may be operated.

e when checking for leaks, the vaporizers should be switched on.

39 The volume of 1 mole of gas

a is equal for all ideal gases at standard temperature and pressure (STP).

b varies with pressure.

c varies with temperature.

d is 22.4 l at room temperature.

e is 1 l at STP.

40 In the event of a failed tracheal intubation in obstetric anaesthesia

a cricoid pressure should be maintained.

b only three attempts at intubation should be made.

c manual lung ventilation should not be attempted.

d the patient should be allowed to awaken.

e isoflurane in oxygen is the safest technique if the operation must proceed.

(Ch. 16, A & S)

a False   The UK standard for oxygen alarms specifies that they are independent of other gas supplies.

b False   Where pipelines are supplied to an anaesthetic machine, they should be disconnected only to ascertain the integrity of the supply from the gas outlet to the Rotameter block, as in the single hose test.

c False   On older anaesthetic machines, an interlock prevented the concurrent use of trichloroethylene and the circle system; on modern machines, this is not so.

d True   The oxygen flush emits gas at a pressure of 400 kPa. This pressure applied to the back bar would cause damage to the Rotameter block, and in order to prevent this a pressure relief valve operating at 35 kPa is inserted downstream of the vaporizers.

e True   This reveals failure to mount vaporizers correctly on the back bar, or failure to close filling caps.

(Ch. 15, A & S)

a True   This is an extension of Avogadro's hypothesis.

b True   The volume of the gas varies inversely with pressure at constant temperature – Boyle's law.

c True   The volume varies directly with the absolute temperature at constant pressure – Charles' law.

d False   The molar volume of all perfect gases is 22.4 l at STP.

e False   See **d** above.

(Ch. 32, A & S)

a True   The risk of regurgitation persists.

b False   However, repeated attempts at intubation by the inexperienced may be dangerous.

c False   Manual ventilation with 100% oxygen may be necessary.

d True   Unless the situation is urgent. Time is required for the anaesthetist to summon help. Regional anaesthesia may also be considered.

e False   Spontaneous ventilation using the agent with which the anaesthetist is most familiar is the preferred technique.

41 **The following anaesthetics may form explosive mixtures when used during the course of a normal anaesthetic:**
a cyclopropane.

b halothane.

c enflurane.

d methoxyflurane.

e diethyl ether.

42 **The combination of atrial fibrillation and tachycardia may indicate**
a uncontrolled thyrotoxicosis.

b digoxin toxicity.

c ventricular bigeminy with escape beats.
d hyperkalaemia.

e hypokalaemia.

43 **Malignant hyperthermia is treated specifically with**
a dantrolene.
b chlorpromazine.
c sodium calcium edetate.
d danthron.
e Ca^{++}.

44 **Compliance**
a of the lung alone is greater than the compliance of the lung and chest together.

b may be measured only during controlled ventilation in the case of dynamic compliance.
c varies directly with age in adults.

d is greater when supine.

e increases during prolonged anaesthesia.

(Ch. 8, A & S)

a **True**   Cyclopropane forms an explosive mixture with oxygen and with nitrous oxide, throughout the range of anaesthetic concentrations.

b **False**   This is non-flammable and non-explosive at atmospheric pressure.

c **False**   This is non-explosive in clinical concentrations in oxygen or in nitrous oxide.

d **False**   This is non-flammable in ordinary clinical use, but burns at higher concentrations and temperatures.

e **True**   Ether is flammable at concentrations greater than 2%. It is essential to avoid diathermy whilst using ether.

(Ch. 3, D)

a **True**   This is an important cause of atrial fibrillation, particularly in the elderly.

b **False**   Bradycardia and ventricular ectopic beats are more common with digoxin toxicity.

c **False**   This may be a manifestation of digoxin toxicity.

d **False**   Ventricular fibrillation may occur in the later stages of hyperkalaemia.

e **True**   If this is severe, atrial tachycardia may produce a reduction in cardiac output.

(Ch. 22, A & S)

a **True**   This is the only specific treatment for malignant hyperpyrexia.

b **False**

c **False**   This is used as a chelating agent in the treatment of poisoning.

d **False**   This is used in the treatment of constipation *(Ch. 1, BNF)*.

e **False**

(Ch. 1, A & S)

a **True**   The reciprocal of total respiratory compliance is equal to the sum of the reciprocals of each of its constituent parts, that is, lungs and chest wall. Therefore lung compliance must be greater than total compliance.

b **False**   Dynamic compliance may be measured during spontaneous ventilation.

c **False**   There is no relationship between compliance and age in healthy subjects.

d **False**   In the supine position, the weight of the chest wall tends to reduce the value of total compliance.

e **False**   During prolonged anaesthesia, lung compliance tends to decrease but may be restored with a large tidal breath.

45 The following drug interactions occur:

a Aspirin displaces warfarin from plasma-protein binding sites.

b Digoxin is more toxic in the presence of hyperkalaemia.

c Vecuronium precipitates in thiopentone.

d Probenecid enhances the actions of penicillin.

e Morphine delays the absorption of paracetamol.

46 In the normal ECG

a there is a Q wave in V_6.

b there is an upright T wave in aVR.

c the S wave is of greater amplitude than the R wave in V_1.

d the PR interval is 0.24 s.

e depolarization lasts 200 ms.

47 A depolarizing block may be produced by

a neostigmine.

b suxamethonium.

c atracurium.

d edrophonium.

e gallamine.

48 Pressure

a equals force × distance.

b equals force per unit area.

c is the rate of doing work.

d can be measured using a column of mercury.

e is measured in newtons.

(Appendix 1, BNF)

a **True** Aspirin (in common with other NSAIDs) prolongs the prothrombin time in patients receiving warfarin.

b **False** Hypokalaemia increases the likelihood of toxicity with digoxin *(Ch. 13, A & S).*

c **True** This is an important interaction, as precipitation may occur in a cannula injection port when vecuronium follows the injection of thiopentone.

d **True** Probenecid is excreted by the kidney in preference to penicillin *(Ch. 10, BNF).*

e **True** Morphine delays gastric emptying.

(Ch. 3, D)

a **True** This represents depolarization of the interventricular septum.

b **False** Repolarization, represented by the T wave, takes place in the opposite direction from that of the major component of the QRS complex.

c **True** V_1 is a right-side lead and ventricular depolarization, represented by the S wave, is directed away from the lead.

d **False** This represents first degree heart block; the upper limit of normal is 0.2 s.

e **True** This is much shorter than the duration of depolarization in skeletal muscle *(Ch. 2, A & S).*

(Ch. 11, A & S)

a **True** Although neostigmine is used usually to antagonize neuromuscular block, high doses of neostigmine may lead to a cholinergic block (as in myasthenia gravis) with a depolarizing characteristic.

b **True**

c **False** This is a non-depolarizing (competitive) agent.

d **False** Theoretically, it should be possible for overdosage with edrophonium to cause a cholinergic block, but its transient action makes this unlikely.

e **False** This is a non-depolarizing agent.

(Ch. 15, A & S)

a **False** Work is defined as the product of force and distance.

b **True** *(Appendix Ib, A & S)*

c **False** Power is defined as the rate of working.

d **True** Hence the use of a mercury barometer and a sphygmomanometer.

e **False** The SI unit of pressure is the pascal (Pa) *(Appendix Ib, A & S).*

49 **The following are true of a supraclavicular approach, in comparison with an axillary approach, to brachial plexus block:**
a There is a greater risk of intravascular injection.

b Analgesia of the shoulder is poorer.
c It is more likely to fail to block the posterior interosseous nerve.

d It is less likely to give analgesia of the forearm.

e There is increased incidence of pneumothorax.

50 **Pain occurs commonly following i.v. injection of**
a thiopentone.

b etomidate.

c suxamethonium.

d neostigmine.

e methohexitone.

51 **Concentrations of the following ions are higher in intracellular fluid than in plasma:**
a potassium.

b sodium.
c phosphate.

d bicarbonate.

e protein.

52 **The following local anaesthetics cause vasoconstriction:**
a lignocaine.
b cocaine.

c amethocaine.

d procaine.

e prilocaine.

(Ch. 25, A & S)

a **False** Intravascular injection commonly complicates the axillary approach.
b **False** Neither approach provides analgesia of the shoulder.
c **False** This is a branch of the radial nerve and is blocked by both techniques.
d **False** The axillary approach is more likely to be associated with this problem.
e **True** The incidence approaches 6%.

(Ch. 9, A & S)

a **False** Pain may occur with thiopentone, but is rare unless small veins and rapid injection are used.
b **True** This occurs in up to 80% of patients. It may be reduced by increasing the speed of injection.
c **False** Suxamethonium is given following induction of anaesthesia, and complaint of pain should not be encountered!
d **False** Pain on injection is not a feature of the use of neostigmine, either for antagonism of neuromuscular block or for treatment of supraventricular tachycardia.
e **True** This has an incidence of up to 21%. It may be minimized by the use of a large vein and by analgesic premedication.

(Ch. 3, A & S)

a **True** Potassium is the main cation in the intracellular compartment, with a concentration of approximately 150 mmol/l.
b **False** Sodium is the principal extracellular cation.
c **True** Intracellular phosphates in the form of ATP and AMP are part of messenger systems in the cell.
d **False** Bicarbonate is primarily an extracellular anion which has roles in buffering and CO_2 transport.
e **False** Intracellular protein anions are present in a concentration lower than that in the plasma.

(Ch. 14, A & S)

a **False**
b **True** This causes vasoconstriction. It is used for this purpose in ENT surgery.
c **False** This has no vasoconstrictor properties. It is used for topical anaesthesia in ophthalmology.
d **False** This causes vasodilatation; for this reason adrenaline is generally added to solutions of procaine.
e **False**

53 Successful ulnar nerve block at the elbow results in
a numbness in the dorsal aspect of the little finger.

b numbness in the whole of the dorsum of the hand.
c paralysis of all the muscles of the thenar eminence.

d numbness of the medial aspect of the forearm.

e neuroma formation, if injection is made into the intercondylar groove.

54 Physical dependence may be produced by
a phenylbutazone.
b pentazocine.

c morphine.
d buprenorphine.

e diazepam.

55 The burned patient
a may develop a high blood concentration of carbon monoxide.

b hypoventilates in the early phase of injury.
c requires i.v. fluid therapy when the burn area is > 15%.
d requires i.v. fluid replacement, given totally as albumin solution.

e should not receive suxamethonium in the acute phase.

56 Trimetaphan
a is a competitive antagonist.

b is a parasympathetic ganglion blocker.
c causes miosis.
d causes depression of respiration.
e is safe in asthmatics.

(Ch. 25, A & S)

a **True** The sensory distribution of the ulnar nerve is to the medial one-and-a-half fingers.

b **False** See **a** above.

c **False** Ulnar nerve block results in paralysis of the hypothenar muscles and adductor pollicis.

d **False** The medial aspect of the forearm is supplied by the medial cutaneous nerve of the forearm, which arises from the brachial plexus.

e **True** Compression of the nerve may be produced by injection of local anaesthetic at this site. It is advisable to inject at a point approximately 2–3 cm proximal to the medial epicondyle.

(Ch. 18, D)

a **False**

b **True** Pentazocine is an opioid analgesic with agonist/antagonist properties, and physical dependence is well recognized with this agent. It is a controlled drug (Schedule 3, Misuse of Drugs Regulations 1985).

c **True** Morphine is a controlled (Schedule 2) drug.

d **True** Buprenorphine is a controlled (Schedule 3) drug, which is subject to 'safe custody' regulations *(BNF)*.

e **True** Physical dependence has been reported with the benzodiazepines.

(Ch. 35, A & S)

a **True** This is the result of inhaling gaseous products of combustion. Carbon monoxide has a high affinity for haemoglobin. High concentrations in burned patients lead to tissue hypoxia.

b **False** The acute response to stress leads to hyperventilation.

c **True** In children, i.v. fluids are required if the burn area is > 10%.

d **False** 50% of i.v. fluid replacement should be given as albumin solution.

e **False** Suxamethonium is hazardous in the later period, between approximately 1 week and 3 months.

(Ch. 36, A & S)

a **True** It acts by competing for acetylcholine receptor sites at the autonomic ganglia.

b **True** It is a sympathetic and parasympathetic ganglion blocker.

c **False** Mydriasis occurs after administration of trimetaphan.

d **False**

e **False** It releases histamine and this limits its use.

57 **The critical temperature of a gas is the temperature**

a   at which latent heat of vaporization is zero.

b   at which latent heat of vaporization is maximum.

c   at which it solidifies.

d   at which it liquefies when critical pressure is applied.

e   above which the gas cannot liquefy, however high the pressure.

58 **Atrial tachycardia with atrioventricular (AV) block**

a   has a ventricular rate of 140–220 beats/min.

b   may be caused by digoxin overdose.

c   may be converted to sinus rhythm by intravenous metoprolol.

d   is unlikely to occur in an otherwise healthy heart.

e   may be treated successfully with i.v. digoxin.

59 **Bronchospasm during anaesthesia may be treated with**

a   aminophylline.

b   salbutamol.

c   ether.

d   metoprolol.

e   sodium cromoglycate.

60 **The Magill attachment**

a   is an example of a Mapleson E system.

b   is functionally similar to the Lack system.

c   is economical in terms of fresh gas flow (FGF) rate when used for IPPV (intermittent positive-pressure ventilation).

d   for spontaneous respiration needs a FGF rate of > 70 ml/kg.

e   can be used for children weighing > 25 kg.

(Ch. 15, A & S)

a **False** Critical temperature is that temperature above which it is not possible to liquefy a gas, even with infinite pressure.
b **False** See **a** above.
c **False** See **a** above.
d **True** The gas in equilibrium with its liquid in this case is strictly termed a vapour.
e **True**

(Ch. 3, D)

a **True** The rate may be slowed by carotid sinus massage.
b **True** This may indicate the need for treatment with a beta-blocker.
c **True** See above.
d **True** In contrast to paroxysmal atrial tachycardia without AV block.
e **True** Digoxin may be used to control the ventricular rate; however, AV block may occur as a toxic effect of digoxin therapy.

(Ch. 22, A & S)

a **True** This is given slowly i.v. in a dose of 250–500 mg.
b **True** This is a specific β_2-adrenoceptor agonist.
c **True** Ether has sympathomimetic actions and has been used to treat bronchospasm during anaesthesia.
d **False** This is a selective beta$_1$-blocker *(Ch. 12, A & S)*.
e **False** Sodium cromoglycate may be used therapeutically for prophylaxis against histamine release, but not for direct treatment.

(Ch. 16, A & S)

a **False** It is described by Mapleson as an 'A' system – the Mapleson E system is represented by the Ayre's T-piece.
b **True** The Lack system is a coaxial version of the Magill attachment, but is not as efficient.
c **False** High FGF rates are required to obviate carbon dioxide rebreathing when this system is used for IPPV.

d **True** This figure is derived from the expected alveolar minute ventilation.
e **True** This is the lower limit of weight for the use of this system.

6. Examination 2

1   Plasma cholinesterase
   a   is manufactured in the liver.
   b   cleaves the amide bond of suxamethonium.

   c   is absent in homozygotes for atypical cholinesterase.

   d   absence is treated with fresh frozen plasma (FFP).

   e   is reduced in concentration by haemofiltration.

2   The following statements are correct:
   a   Acidosis associated with diabetic coma is caused by vomiting.

   b   Acidosis associated with diarrhoea is caused by loss of base.

   c   Acidosis during renal failure is caused by decreased sodium excretion.
   d   Metabolic alkalosis may be reversed with i.v. saline.

   e   When blood is taken from a patient at 32°C, the measured Pa_{CO2} is higher when the sample is analysed at 37°C.

(Ch. 11, A & S)

a	**True**	This is one of the proteins synthesized by the liver.
b	**False**	There is no amide bond in suxamethonium, which comprises two molecules of acetylcholine joined by an ester link.
c	**False**	Patients who are homozygous for the atypical enzyme do not metabolize suxamethonium at a normal rate, but the concentration of plasma cholinesterase may be normal.
d	**False**	Treatment in such patients involves maintenance of ventilation and anaesthesia while spontaneous metabolism occurs. FFP is not warranted in this situation.
e	**False**	Its concentration is reduced by plasmapheresis. Haemofiltration should have no effect.

a	**False**	It is caused by accumulation of ketone bodies as a result of increased lipolysis *(Ch. 8, D)*.
b	**False**	Alkalosis is more usual, secondary to hypokalaemia. Acidosis may be a manifestation of circulatory insufficiency *(Ch. 21, A & S)*.
c	**False**	Acidosis is caused by inability to excrete hydrogen ions *(Ch. 6, D)*.
d	**True**	This is the initial treatment of infants with pyloric stenosis, because the additional chloride ions permit renal excretion of bicarbonate *(Ch. 9, D)*.
e	**True**	Gas solubility is increased at lower temperatures *(Ch. 15, A & S)*.

3   Bupivacaine is
a   highly protein-bound.
b   lipid-soluble.

c   a cause of methaemoglobinaemia.

d   suitable for continuous epidural anaesthesia.

e   highly cardiotoxic.

---

4   The following are true of gas cylinders:
a   Oxygen is supplied in cylinders at a pressure of 120 lb/in^2.

b   Nitrous oxide is supplied at a pressure of 44 lb/in^2.

c   Full nitrous oxide cylinders contain only liquid nitrogen.
d   Nitrous oxide cylinders should not be stored below –7°C.

e   Helium cylinders are coloured pink.

---

5   Enhanced neuromuscular blockade occurs with the following combinations:
a   suxamethonium and neostigmine.

b   tubocurarine and ecothiopate.

c   vecuronium and tobramycin.

d   rocuronium and atropine.

e   vecuronium and isoflurane.

(Ch. 14, A & S)

a **True** 95% of bupivacaine in blood is bound to protein.
b **True** In common with all local anaesthetic agents, bupivacaine is lipid-soluble.
c **False** Bupivacaine has not been associated with methaemoglobinaemia – this complication is usually ascribed to prilocaine.
d **True** Bupivacaine is the agent of choice for continuous epidural anaesthesia.
e **True** Bupivacaine is amongst the most cardiotoxic of all the local anaesthetic agents.

(Ch. 16, A & S)

a **False** The usual pressure in a full oxygen cylinder is 13.7 MPa – approximately 2000 lb/in^2.
b **False** Nitrous oxide cylinders are supplied usually with a pressure of 44 bar (750 lb/in^2 – 4.5 MPa).
c **False** Nitrous oxide cylinders contain liquid nitrous oxide!
d **True** All gas cylinders for medical use should be stored in a warm dry place and not subjected to extremes of temperature. –7°C is the pseudo-critical temperature for Entonox.
e **False** Helium cylinders are brown.

(Ch. 11, A & S)

a **True** One of the characteristics of a depolarizing block is that an anticholinesterase (such as neostigmine) may make the block more intense.
b **False** Ecothiopate depresses plasma cholinesterase. There is no interaction with a non-depolarizing drug, such as curare.
c **True** The intraperitoneal administration of aminoglycoside antibiotics may prolong the effect of non-depolarizing neuromuscular blockers.
d **False** The anti-muscarinic actions of atropine have no influence on neuromuscular blocking drugs.
e **True** The use of inhalational anaesthetics, especially isoflurane and enflurane, prolongs the neuromuscular blockade induced by non-depolarizing agents.

6 **Administration of sevoflurane**
a requires use of a specialized vaporizer.
b results in more rapid recovery than with desflurane.
c causes myocardial depression.
d potentiates the action of neuromuscular relaxants.
e is contraindicated in infants.

7 **During one-lung ventilation**
a a double-lumen bronchial tube is required.

b increased intrapulmonary shunting results in decreased Pa_{O_2}.
c increased intrapulmonary shunting results in decreased Sa_{O_2}.
d increased intrapulmonary shunting results in increased Pa_{CO_2}.

e an $F_{I_{O_2}}$ of 0.6 or greater is necessary.

8 **In a patient who has received alpha-adrenoceptor blockers, the following would be expected:**
a cold skin.
b miosis.

c decreased arterial pressure.
d orthostatic hypotension.

e bradycardia.

9 **A 2.5% solution of thiopentone injected intra-arterially causes fewer problems than a 5% solution because**
a less microcrystals and microaggregates are formed.

b it is less alkaline.

c it is isotonic, whereas the 5% solution is hypertonic.
d the pH of the 2.5% solution is neutral.
e it is more easily dispersed in the arterial blood.

(Ch. 8, A & S)

a	**False**	Its physical properties permit the use of a standard vaporizer.
b	**False**	Recovery is slower than with desflurane.
c	**False**	At clinical concentrations its effects are slight.
d	**True**	To a similar extent to other volatile agents.
e	**False**	It is a useful agent for inhalational induction of anaesthesia.

(Ch. 38, A & S)

a	**True**	In theory, single-lumen tubes may be employed, but a double-lumen tube is the commonest type used for this purpose.
b	**True**	Shunting occurs through the non-ventilated lung.
c	**True**	Decreased saturation accompanies the decrease in Pa_{O_2}.
d	**False**	Carbon dioxide excretion is relatively unaffected by one-lung ventilation.
e	**False**	Inspired oxygen concentration in excess of 60% does not increase oxygen delivery, and may negate the useful effect of hypoxic pulmonary vasoconstriction.

(Ch. 12, A & S)

a	**False**	Alpha-adrenoceptor blockade results in peripheral vasodilatation.
b	**True**	The sympathetic supply to the pupil via alpha-adrenoceptors produces pupillary dilation.
c	**True**	Peripheral vasoconstrictor tone is reduced with alpha-blockade.
d	**True**	The normal physiological response on assuming the upright posture is peripheral vasoconstriction mediated via alpha-adrenoceptors.
e	**False**	The chronotropic supply to the heart is mediated via beta-adrenoceptors.

(Ch. 9, A & S)

a	**True**	Crystal formation is thought to be related to the concentration of solution, and thus the 2.5% solution is safer.
b	**False**	The pH of a solution (whether 2.5% or 5%) of thiopentone is 10.5.
c	**False**	The tonicity of the fluid is not the limiting factor in this case.
d	**False**	See **b** above.
e	**False**	See **a** above.

10 **An increase in minute volume may be caused by**

a increased CSF H^+ concentration.

b Pa_{O_2} of 8 kPa.

c a chronic anaemia of Hb 5 g/dl.

d i.v. adrenaline.

e breathing 0.03% CO_2 in air.

---

11 **The following are complications of gallstones:**

a pancreatitis.

b cholangitis.

c hiatus hernia.

d intestinal obstruction.

e carcinoma of the gall bladder.

---

12 **Rate of gastric emptying is diminished by the following drugs in therapeutic dosage:**

a atropine.

b morphine.

c apomorphine.

d codeine.

e neostigmine.

(Ch. 1, A & S)

a True This is the normal physiological mechanism whereby central chemoreceptor stimulation results in an increase in minute volume.

b False Peripheral hypoxic stimulation increases minute volume only if Pa_{O_2} is less than 8 kPa in the presence of a normal Pa_{CO_2}.

c False In chronic anaemia, there is a compensatory increase in 2,3-diphosphoglycerate (2,3-DPG), concentration in the red cell, and tissue oxygenation is impaired less than in acute anaemia *(Ch. 6, A & S)*.

d True Exogenous catecholamine stimulation of the cardiovascular and respiratory systems occurs.

e False 0.03% CO_2 is the normal value for concentration of carbon dioxide in air.

(Ch. 10, D)

a True There is a frequent association between disease of the biliary tract and pancreatitis.

b True

c False This is not a complication of cholelithiasis, although the two conditions may coexist.

d True A large gallstone may reach the intestinal tract and cause obstruction, usually at the terminal ileum.

e False Carcinoma of the gall bladder is very uncommon, whereas gallstones are present in 15–20% of the adult population, the frequency being greater than 40% in those over 60 years of age.

(Ch. 7, A & S)

a True Atropine is an anticholinergic and therefore inhibits gastrointestinal motility.

b True This has a profound inhibitory effect upon the rate of gastric emptying; this is not antagonized by metoclopramide.

c False This induces vomiting and therefore increases the rate of gastric emptying!

d True This inhibits gastrointestinal motility.

e False This does not delay gastric emptying.

13 If surgery is required in a patient who has suffered myocardial infarction complicated by heart failure

  a there is at least a tenfold increase in the risk of reinfarction if surgery occurs within 3–6 months of a previous myocardial infarction.

  b hypotension is desirable during anaesthesia, to reduce cardiac work.

  c no opioid premedication should be given.

  d tracheal intubation should be undertaken only during a light plane of anaesthesia.

  e halothane should be avoided.

14 Irrigation of the bladder during surgery for TURP (transurethral resection of the prostate) may result in

  a hyponatraemia.

  b haemodilution.

  c haemolysis.

  d hyperkalaemia.

  e hypercalcaemia.

15 Dependence on opioids

  a is always associated with tolerance.

  b results in tolerance to barbiturates.

  c increases the risk of acquisition of hepatitis.

  d may be treated with oral methadone.

  e may be treated with an opioid antagonist.

16 In the infant undergoing general anaesthesia

  a the larynx is placed higher in the neck than in the adult.

  b the use of the Macintosh laryngoscope is recommended.

  c the tracheal tube should be age/4 + 4.5 mm internal diameter.

  d preformed tracheal tubes avoid bronchial intubation.

  e a praecordial stethoscope provides an index of cardiac output.

(Ch. 40, A & S)

a **True** Within 3–6 months of myocardial infarction, the risk of reinfarction is approximately 16%.

b **False** Maintenance of normotension is desirable during anaesthesia; hypotension reduces coronary blood flow if the arteries are stenosed.
c **False** Premedication should be sufficient to allay anxiety.
d **False** Sufficient anaesthesia is required to mitigate the response associated with tracheal intubation.
e **False** Small concentrations of halothane may be beneficial by depressing myocardial oxygen consumption.

(Ch. 26, A & S)

a **True** Dilutional hyponatraemia may occur because of absorption of irrigation fluid into venous sinuses.
b **True** Haemodilution and reduction in haematocrit may indicate absorption of large volumes of fluid.
c **False** Haemolysis is not a feature of dilutional hyponatraemia.
d **False** Absorption of irrigating solution does not cause an increase in serum potassium concentration.
e **False** Calcium is not a constituent of bladder-irrigating solutions.

(Ch. 18, D; Ch. 4, BNF)

a **False** Dependence and tolerance are separate entities. Acute tolerance may occur without dependence, but tolerance may occur also as a consequence of dependence.
b **False** Cross-tolerance does not occur, but enzyme inducers, e.g. ethyl alcohol, may result in tolerance to i.v. barbiturates.
c **True** As a result of needle contamination.
d **True** This is an opioid agonist.
e **True** A withdrawal syndrome is provoked.

(Ch. 33, A & S)

a **True** The larynx is at C3–4 compared with C5–6 in the adult.
b **False** Laryngoscopy is easier with a straight-bladed laryngoscope.
c **False** The size required is age/4 + 4 mm.
d **False** Preformed tubes of fixed length may result in bronchial intubation.
e **True** In the infant, the intensity of sound varies with the stroke volume.

17 **Infrared gas analysis is a suitable technique for the measurement of clinical concentrations of**

a oxygen.

b nitrous oxide.

c CO_2.

d helium.

e ethyl alcohol.

---

18 **Increased serum urea concentration after a large haematemesis may be caused by**

a dehydration.

b potassium loss.
c metabolic acidosis.

d depressed renal function.
e increased protein catabolism in the gut.

---

19 **Ethanol causes**

a enzyme induction in the liver.

b vasodilatation in skin.
c antagonism of respiratory depression caused by barbiturates.

d direct liver cell damage.

e peripheral neuropathy.

---

20 **Ventricular ectopic beats**

a may be differentiated from atrial fibrillation by inspection of the peripheral pulse.
b may precipitate ventricular fibrillation after myocardial infarction.

c are associated with digoxin toxicity.
d are a good indicator of ischaemic heart disease.
e may be treated with verapamil.

(Ch. 20, A & S)

a   **False**   Oxygen concentrations may be measured by paramagnetic, polarographic, or fuel cell analysis, by mass spectrometry or chemically. Infrared analysis is not suitable.

b   **True**   Nitrous oxide has a peak absorption at 3.9 μm, which is well within the infrared spectrum. When infrared gas analysis is used to measure end-expired CO_2, there may be interference from nitrous oxide.

c   **True**   This is the Luft principle, described first in 1943 and employed routinely in capnography.

d   **False**   Helium is an inert gas and does not have a suitable absorption spectrum in the infrared range.

e   **True**   An infrared vapour analyser can be used to measure expired ethyl alcohol concentration.

(Ch. 7, D)

a   **True**   Dehydration results from movement of interstitial fluid into the circulation to replace the lost blood.

b   **False**   This is not a feature of this condition.

c   **False**   The serum urea concentration is not influenced by acid–base abnormalities.

d   **True**   Blood loss and hypotension may result in renal failure.

e   **True**

(Ch. 18, D)

a   **True**   Microsomal enzyme induction may occur with chronic alcohol abuse.

b   **True**   Ethanol is a potent peripheral vasodilator.

c   **False**   Ethanol is a CNS depressant and does not reverse depression caused by other CNS depressants.

d   **False**   Unlike chloroform, ethanol does not cause direct liver cell damage.

e   **True**   This may occur in the alcoholic because of nutritional deficiency *(Ch. 12, D)*.

(Ch. 3, D)

a   **False**   An ECG is required for accurate diagnosis.

b   **True**   This is more likely if an ectopic beat coincides with the T wave of the previous complex.

c   **True**   Bigeminy is common.

d   **False**   Ventricular ectopic beats may occur in normal individuals.

e   **False**   The main indication for verapamil is supraventricular tachycardia.

21 **Intermittent positive pressure ventilation (IPPV) in the anaesthetized patient results in**

a decreased functional residual capacity (FRC).

b increased lung compliance.

c increased intrapleural pressure.
d decreased cardiac output in hypovolaemia.

e increased right atrial pressure.

---

22 **The risk of fire in the operating room may be reduced by**
a connecting trolleys by a high resistance to the floor.

b avoiding battery-operated equipment whenever possible.

c the use of an isolation transformer.

d use of footwear with a resistance of 10 000 ohms.

e siting electrical sockets higher than 1.5 m above the floor.

---

23 **FFP**
a must be crossmatched.

b may be used to treat DIC (disseminated intravascular coagulation).
c is used during massive blood transfusion.

d is indicated in the treatment of burns.

e is indicated in the treatment of renal failure.

(Ch. 1, A & S)

a	**True**	FRC is reduced during anaesthesia to a similar extent by either IPPV or spontaneous ventilation.
b	**False**	Lung compliance remains unchanged, or may decrease if a low tidal volume (VT) is employed.
c	**True**	IPPV increases intrapleural pressure during inspiration.
d	**True**	The increased intrapulmonary and intrathoracic pressures reduce venous return to the heart, especially in the hypovolaemic patient, and this results in a decreased cardiac output *(Ch. 2, A & S)*.
e	**True**	Increased intrathoracic pressure is transmitted to the great vessels and right atrium.

(Ch. 15, A & S)

a	**True**	Trolleys are connected to the floor by a high resistance. This prevents the accumulation of static electrical charges, whilst maintaining electrical isolation for mains voltages (240 V r.m.s.).
b	**False**	Such equipment is recommended because the low voltage employed reduces the risk of sparks.
c	**True**	An isolation transformer reduces the risk of electrocution, but not of spark formation.
d	**False**	Footwear designed for use in the operating theatre should have a resistance of greater than 1 Mohm.
e	**True**	Most inflammable vapours are heavier than air.

a	**False**	Rhesus compatibility is not required but it must be ABO compatible.
b	**True**	FFP is rich in heat-labile coagulation factors.
c	**True**	Massive blood transfusion may lead to dilutional coagulopathy. This is treated with FFP, platelets and, sometimes, factor VIII concentrate *(Ch. 31, A & S)*.
d	**True**	Burns produce a rapid loss of plasma protein, including the plasma coagulation factors which are present in FFP *(Ch. 35, A & S)*.
e	**False**	There is no specific indication for using FFP in renal failure.

24   Suxamethonium

a   must be stored below 4°C.

b   causes a reduction in intracellular potassium concentration.

c   increases intraocular pressure because of an increase in venous pressure.

d   has a prolonged action in liver failure.

e   is contraindicated in severe burns.

---

25   Which of the following measurements are satisfactory for assessing adequate recovery of neuromuscular function?

a   minute volume.

b   generation of a vital capacity of 10 ml/kg.

c   head-lift sustained for 5 s.

d   tidal volume (VT).

e   respiratory rate.

---

26   An obese patient is more likely than a normal patient to demonstrate

a   difficulty of tracheal intubation.

b   hypoxaemia.

c   abnormal sensitivity to muscle relaxants.

d   abnormal sensitivity to thiopentone.

e   hypertension.

(Ch. 11, A & S)

a **True** Some deterioration occurs if it is stored above this temperature.
b **True** This is associated with an increase in extracellular potassium concentration.
c **True** The increase in intraocular pressure caused by suxamethonium is caused partly by an increase in venous pressure. Contraction of the tonic fibres of extraocular muscles is also contributory.
d **True** Plasma cholinesterase concentration is decreased in the presence of hepatic failure.
e **True** Hyperkalaemia is particularly marked in patients with severe burns or extensive muscle damage, recently paraplegic patients, and patients with peripheral neuropathies.

(Ch. 23, A & S)

a **False** This is not a reliable measure of recovery, as normal values may be achieved during partial paralysis.
b **True**
c **True** This indicates absence of fade.
d **False** Although this may be adequate whilst neuromuscular recovery is incomplete, it indicates that recovery is occurring.
e **False** Respiratory rate depends upon respiratory drive, and is independent of neuromuscular transmission.

(Ch. 40, A & S)

a **True** In the morbidly obese, direct laryngoscopy may be difficult to perform.
b **True** This occurs because of a decrease in FRC and increase in airway closure.
c **False** Abnormal sensitivity does not exist. However, if drugs are given on a body weight basis, overdosage may result.
d **False** See **c** above.
e **True** But care should be taken not to overestimate arterial pressure because an inappropriately small sphygmomanometer cuff is used.

27 The Bain system
a cannot be sterilized.
b is a variant of the Mapleson A breathing system.
c is dangerous if the inner tube becomes disconnected at the patient end.
d has tubing of > 1 m in length.

e should be used with a fresh gas flow (FGF) equal to minute volume during spontaneous ventilation.

28 Reduction in blood glucose concentration is caused by
a isoprenaline.
b phenformin.

c tolbutamide.

d hydrocortisone.
e alpha-adrenergic blocking agents.

29 A serum potassium concentration of 2.5 mmol/l and serum bicarbonate concentration of 15 mmol/l are compatible with
a treatment of diabetic ketoacidosis with insulin alone.
b primary hyperaldosteronism.
c transfusion of a large volume of blood.
d pyloric stenosis.
e failure of ventilation in chronic bronchitis.

30 Dilatation of the cervix may result in
a laryngospasm.
b tachycardia.
c bradycardia.
d postoperative shivering.
e intense bleeding.

(Ch. 16, A & S)

a **False** The components of the Bain system may be sterilized by heat.
b **False** It is a variant of the Mapleson D system.
c **False** Disconnection at the machine end is dangerous, as it results in rebreathing of carbon dioxide.
d **True** The volume of the tubing must be greater than the patient's tidal volume. 1 m of 22-mm tubing has a volume of about 600 ml.
e **False** FGF rate should be two to three times the minute volume to prevent rebreathing during spontaneous ventilation *(Appendix VII, A & S)*.

(Ch. 8, D)

a **False** Isoprenaline is a β-1 adrenergic agonist.
b **True** Phenformin is a biguanide oral hypoglycaemic agent with a strong propensity to cause lactic acidosis. Metformin is the only biguanide now available.
c **True** Tolbutamide is a sulphonylurea hypoglycaemic agent with a short duration of action.
d **False** Steroids tend to promote glycogenolysis and gluconeogenesis.
e **False** Alpha-adrenoceptor blockers act on peripheral receptors and have no pancreatic action.

(Ch. 21, A & S; Ch. 5, D)

a **True** But metabolic acidosis may result in hyperkalaemia.
b **False** Metabolic alkalosis usually accompanies potassium depletion.
c **False** This may produce transient hyperkalaemia.
d **False** This usually causes alkalosis.
e **False** This may result in compensated respiratory acidosis: the serum bicarbonate concentration would be elevated.

(Ch. 26, A & S)

a **True** This may occur under light anaesthesia.
b **False** Bradycardia is the usual response.
c **True** Because of insufficient depth of anaesthesia.
d **False** This is associated with excessive use of volatile agents.
e **False**

31   In day-case anaesthesia
a   tracheal intubation is contraindicated.

b   ketamine is a useful agent.

c   after circumcision under caudal analgesia, micturition is often delayed.

d   patients may be permitted to drive or operate machinery after 12 h.

e   thiopentone is not contraindicated for induction.

---

32   Which of the following would lead you to postpone routine surgery or modify your anaesthetic technique?
a   glycosuria on routine testing.

b   haemoglobin concentration of 10.8 g/dl.

c   bilirubinaemia.

d   white cell count of 8.0×10^9/l.

e   serum potassium concentration of 2.5 mmol/l.

---

33   The following may be compressed together safely in a cylinder:
a   helium and oxygen.

b   ethylene and oxygen.

c   nitrous oxide and oxygen.

d CO_2 and oxygen.

e   oxygen and acetylene.

(Ch. 30, A & S)

a **False** Provided that patients are supervised closely in the early postoperative period, there is no contraindication to tracheal intubation.

b **False** Dysphoric reactions, emergence phenomena and prolonged recovery preclude the usefulness of ketamine in this situation.

c **True** This is a common occurrence.

d **False** A minimum of 24 h is required.

e **True** Although slightly larger doses than normal may be necessary, because premedication is usually omitted.

(Ch. 18, A & S)

a **True** This is not a reliable test of diabetes mellitus, but would be an indication for further investigation.

b **False** A haemoglobin concentration of 10 g/dl is acceptable for routine surgery.

c **True** Bilirubinaemia is an indication for further investigation to elucidate its origin.

d **False** This is a normal white cell count.

e **True** This represents severe hypokalaemia and should be treated preoperatively.

(Ch. 16, A & S)

a **True** Helium (79%) and oxygen (21%) mixture is available in black cylinders with white and brown quartered shoulders at a pressure of 137 bar.

b **False** Ethylene is explosive. It is unwise to compress explosive gases with oxygen.

c **True** This is available as a 50% mixture as Entonox at a pressure of 137 bar.

d **True** CO_2 and oxygen mixtures are available in black cylinders with white and grey quartered shoulders.

e **False** See **b** above. Oxyacetylene welding equipment derives its supply from separate oxygen and acetylene cylinders.

34   Lignocaine
a   is metabolized by plasma cholinesterases.

b   has a longer duration of action than procaine.

c   is destroyed by first-pass metabolism after oral administration.

d   can pass through mucous membranes.

e   is an ester.

35   Intrathecal morphine produces
a   nausea and vomiting.
b   itching.
c   respiratory depression.

d   muscle weakness.

e   urinary retention.

36   When anaesthetizing a patient after head injury
a   spontaneous ventilation is an acceptable technique.
b   head flexion may increase intracranial pressure (ICP).

c   the patient should be normovolaemic to ensure adequate cerebral blood flow.
d   autoregulation may be impaired when mean arterial pressure (MAP) is < 80 mmHg.

e   opioids must be avoided.

(Ch. 14, A & S)

a **False**   Lignocaine is an amide local anaesthetic agent. It was first synthesized in 1948.
b **True**   Procaine is an ester-linked anaesthetic agent, metabolized by plasma cholinesterase.
c **True**   There is significant metabolism of lignocaine in the liver. It also has a very short plasma half-life.
d **True**   Care has to be taken that the toxic dose of 200 mg for an adult is not exceeded when lignocaine is applied to mucous membranes.
e **False**

(Ch. 10, A & S)

a **True**   These are common side-effects.
b **True**   Especially of the nose.
c **True**   This may be severe and of late onset. It is recommended that after intrathecal administration of morphine, close supervision of the patient's respiration is maintained for at least 12 h.
d **False**   Muscle weakness is not associated with intrathecal morphine alone.
e **True**   This is a distressing side-effect in 90% of males.

(Ch. 37, A & S)

a **False**   Increases in Pa_{CO_2} and ICP are likely to occur.
b **True**   Head flexion may restrict the venous drainage from the cranium and cause an increase in ICP.
c **True**

d **True**   The lower limit of autoregulation is normally 60 mmHg. However, autoregulation may be impaired at a higher arterial pressure in a patient with head injury.
e **False**   There is no reason to avoid opioids provided adequate ventilation is ensured.

37 **The vapour concentration obtained from a Boyle's bottle containing liquid anaesthetic depends upon**
   a specific gravity of the liquid.
   b specific heat of the liquid.

   c saturated vapour pressure of the liquid.
   d latent heat of vaporization of the liquid.

   e gas flow rate.

38 **Digoxin therapy in atrial fibrillation causes**
   a positive inotropic effect.

   b positive chronotropic effect.
   c increase in stroke volume.

   d increased refractory period of ventricular muscle.

   e delayed velocity of conduction in bundle of His.

39 **Angina is a recognized feature of**
   a aortic stenosis.
   b anaemia.

   c polyarthritis.

   d hypothyroidism.

   e paroxysmal supraventricular tachycardia (SVT).

40 **The following arterial blood gas values: Pa_{O_2} 8 kPa; Pa_{CO_2} 4 kPa; pH 7.44; base excess −1 are compatible with**
   a alveolar hypoventilation.
   b compensated metabolic alkalosis.
   c Lorrain-Smith effect.

   d pulmonary atelectasis.
   e 48 h at an altitude of 3500 m.

(Ch. 15, A & S)

a	**False**	Specific gravity has no influence on vapour pressure.
b	**True**	Vaporization is accompanied by a decrease in temperature. Specific heat determines rate of cooling and thus influences saturated vapour pressure.
c	**True**	
d	**True**	Latent heat of vaporization determines the extent of cooling with evaporation. The temperature in turn influences the saturated vapour pressure.
e	**True**	The greater the gas flow, the greater is the total mass of vapour in the final gas mixture. However, at a given bypass setting, an increase in total gas flow rate decreases the delivered concentration.

(Ch. 3, D; Ch. 2, BNF)

a	**True**	But its main effect is to increase the degree of atrioventricular (AV) block and reduce ventricular rate.
b	**False**	The aim of digoxin therapy is to slow the ventricular rate.
c	**True**	As a result of the reduced ventricular rate, ventricular filling is improved and this may result in an increase in stroke volume.
d	**False**	The refractory period is shortened by digoxin therapy; this may result in ventricular tachycardia.
e	**True**	This is an important mechanism in controlling ventricular rate.

(Ch. 3, D)

a	**True**	
b	**True**	It may occur with severe anaemia (< 5 g/dl), especially in older patients *(Ch. 11, D)*.
c	**False**	Although aortic valvular disease may accompany polyarthritis, angina is not normally a feature.
d	**False**	In hypothyroidism the basal metabolic rate is depressed; angina is not a feature.
e	**True**	The increased oxygen demand produced by SVT may sometimes lead to angina.

(Ch. 1, A & S)

a	**False**	Increased Pa_{CO_2} is characteristic of alveolar hypoventilation.
b	**False**	The base excess is positive in metabolic alkalosis *(Ch. 21, A & S)*.
c	**True**	The Lorrain-Smith effect describes pulmonary oxygen toxicity, which may result subsequently in hypoxaemia.
d	**True**	This results in increased pulmonary shunt.
e	**True**	Unacclimatized persons ascending to altitude hyperventilate.

41 **Drugs used in the treatment of organophosphorus poisoning include**
a neostigmine.

b pralidoxime.

c atropine.
d propranolol.
e chlorpromazine.

42 **If helium is substituted for nitrogen in an air mixture, the resultant gas**
a is less dense.

b has a higher solubility in tissues.
c causes hypnosis.
d is more flammable.
e is used during upper airway obstruction.

43 **Administration of quinidine may cause**
a hypertension.

b increased refractory period of ventricular muscle.

c increased stroke volume.
d supraventricular tachycardia.
e circulatory arrest.

44 **The volume of fluid flowing in a laminar fashion through a tube is directly proportional to**
a the density of the fluid.

b the length of the tube.

c the pressure difference across the tube.
d the fourth power of the radius of the tube.
e the viscosity of the fluid.

(Ch. 19, D)

a **False** Organophosphorus compounds are cholinesterase inhibitors; neostigmine would enhance the poisoning.
b **True** Pralidoxime, a cholinesterase reactivator, has an action similar to that of atropine; treatment may need to be repeated every 30 min as necessary.
c **True** See **a** above.
d **False** Propranolol is a beta-adrenergic blocker.
e **False** Chlorpromazine does not possess anticholinergic properties.

(Ch. 15, A & S)

a **True** The density of the mixture of helium is about one-third that of air.
b **False** Helium is less soluble than nitrogen.
c **False** Helium is an inert gas and is not narcotic.
d **False** Helium is not flammable.
e **True** As a result of its lower density, helium/oxygen flows at a greater rate than air during turbulence.

(Ch. 3, D; Ch. 2, BNF)

a **False** Quinidine is a myocardial depressant and may cause hypotension.
b **False** Ventricular conduction is slowed because of slowing of the sodium current across the cell membrane.
c **False** Quinidine is a myocardial depressant.
d **False** This is one of the indications for quinidine therapy.
e **True** As a result of a combination of myocardial and conducting system depression.

(Ch. 15, A & S)

a **False** The density of fluid is a factor governing turbulent flow through an orifice.
b **False** The volume of fluid flow is inversely proportional to the length.
c **True**
d **True**
e **False** Flow is inversely proportional to viscosity.

45 Which of the following are true of the soda lime used in a circle system?
a It should fill at least half of the canister.

b It requires water for CO_2 to be absorbed.
c It may absorb up to 20% of its weight of CO_2.
d It consists mainly of calcium carbonate.

e Its indicator changes from white to pink with use.

---

46 Ketamine should be avoided
a in the presence of increased arterial pressure.

b in pregnancy.
c in shock.

d in the asthmatic.

e in the presence of facial burns.

---

47 Pulse pressure increases with
a moderate increase in total peripheral resistance.
b increased stroke volume.

c atherosclerosis.

d decreased blood viscosity.

e moderate hypercapnia.

---

48 The following occur in vomiting associated with pyloric stenosis:
a alkaline urine.
b hyperchloraemia.
c hypernatraemia.
d acidosis.
e increased blood urea concentration.

(Ch. 16, A & S)

a	**True**	Soda lime should fill the container, but should not be compacted so as to increase respiratory resistance.
b	**True**	The reaction requires the presence of water.
c	**True**	Soda lime can absorb up to 20% of its weight.
d	**False**	The primary constituent (94%) of soda lime is calcium hydroxide.
e	**False**	The indicator in Durasorb changes from pink to white with exhaustion.

(Ch. 9, A & S)

a	**True**	Ketamine has a hypertensive effect and may exacerbate existing hypertension.
b	**False**	
c	**False**	Ketamine has been employed successfully in the field situation for extrication of casualties; prior administration of atropine is recommended as salivation may be stimulated.
d	**False**	Ketamine has been used successfully during status asthmaticus because it causes sympatho-adrenal stimulation.
e	**False**	Ketamine may be a useful agent because the airway reflexes are depressed less than by other agents; prior administration of atropine is recommended.

(Ch. 2, A & S)

a	**True**	
b	**True**	An increase in stroke volume results in increases in systolic arterial pressure and pulse pressure.
c	**True**	In atherosclerosis, the compliance of the arterial vasculature is reduced and pulse pressure increases.
d	**False**	Although the flow of Newtonian fluid is inversely proportional to its viscosity, changes in blood viscosity have no influence on pulse pressure.
e	**True**	This stimulates the myocardium by increasing plasma catecholamines. The resultant increase in cardiac output increases pulse pressure.

(Ch. 9, D)

a	**True**	Alkalosis develops because of loss of hydrogen ions.
b	**False**	Chloride ions are lost in addition to hydrogen ions.
c	**False**	
d	**False**	
e	**True**	Blood urea concentration may be increased because of dehydration.

49 **Dopamine at a rate of 5 μg/kg per min i.v. is likely to result in**
a coronary artery dilatation.

b renal vasodilatation.
c splanchnic vasoconstriction.
d increased aldosterone secretion.
e bradycardia.

50 **Prolonged vomiting causes**
a hypokalaemia.

b decreased serum chloride concentration.
c raised serum urea concentration.
d hypovolaemia.
e increased anion gap.

51 **Clonidine treatment**
a is an indication for preoperative infusion of noradrenaline.

b causes sedation.
c should be discontinued 6 h before surgery.

d may be used to treat sympathetically mediated pain.
e may cause psychiatric depression.

52 **Methaemoglobinaemia**
a may be due to idiosyncrasy to small doses of drugs.

b is followed usually by significant haemolysis.
c may be treated with i.v. methylene blue.

d reduces the oxygen-carrying capacity of blood.

e may be caused by prilocaine.

(Ch. 12, A & S)

a **False** In this dosage, it has a positive inotropic effect but coronary vasodilatation does not occur.
b **True** This is the upper limit of the dose used to dilate renal vessels.
c **False** It usually causes splanchnic vasodilatation.
d **False** There is no effect on aldosterone output.
e **False** Dopamine is a β-agonist and tachycardia is more likely at this infusion rate.

(Ch. 9, D; Ch. 21, A & S)

a **True** Loss of hydrogen ions from the stomach results in metabolic alkalosis. This promotes potassium excretion in the kidney, with resultant hypokalaemia.
b **True** This is caused by loss of hydrochloric acid from the stomach.
c **True** Secondary to dehydration.
d **True** This is the same mechanism as **c** above.
e **False** Increased anion gap is an indication of the presence of ketoacidosis or lactic acidosis.

(Ch. 10, A & S; Ch. 2, BNF)

a **False** It is a centrally acting antihypertensive agent. A noradrenaline infusion is contraindicated.
b **True** This may arise after perioperative use.
c **False** Sudden withdrawal of clonidine may precipitate a hypertensive crisis.
d **True** Clonidine activates alpha$_2$-receptors.
e **True** Depression may be a side-effect of clonidine usage.

(Ch. 14, A & S)

a **False** Methaemoglobinaemia results from oxidation of ferrous to ferric ions in haemoglobin, and requires the presence of a strong oxidizing agent. Idiosyncrasy to drugs does not provide this mechanism.
b **False** This is not a feature of methaemoglobinaemia.
c **True** In a dose of 1 mg/kg this reverses methaemoglobinaemia rapidly.
d **True** Ferric haemoglobin is unable to combine normally with oxygen, thereby reducing oxygen-carrying capacity.
e **True** Prilocaine in a dose exceeding 600 mg may produce methaemoglobinaemia. Fetal haemoglobin is more sensitive and therefore prilocaine is contraindicated during labour.

53 Pulmonary oedema may result from
a tricuspid incompetence.
b left atrial myxoma.

c uncomplicated aortic stenosis.

d myocardial infarction.

e mitral incompetence.

54 Tachycardia occurring immediately after tracheal intubation
a may be produced by suxamethonium.

b may be caused by overdose of thiopentone.

c is accentuated in hypertensive patients.

d may be attenuated by pretreatment with metoprolol.

e may be related to hypoxia.

55 The ulnar nerve supplies
a all interossei muscles.

b the first and second lumbricals.
c opponens pollicis.
d adductor pollicis.

e the skin of the thenar eminence.

56 There is an increased likelihood of convulsions in epileptics treated with
a thiopentone.
b diazepam.
c methohexitone.

d enflurane.

e suxamethonium.

(Ch. 3, D)

a	**False**	
b	**True**	A left atrial myxoma represents an outflow obstruction to the pulmonary circulation. This may increase pulmonary venous pressure and cause pulmonary oedema.
c	**False**	Aortic stenosis in the presence of a competent mitral valve and a healthy myocardium should not result in pulmonary oedema.
d	**True**	Pulmonary oedema is a common complication of severe myocardial infarction.
e	**True**	This is a common accompaniment of mitral valve disease.

(Ch. 22, A & S)

a	**False**	Suxamethonium may cause bradycardia, but usually only after repeated doses.
b	**True**	Overdose of thiopentone may lead to hypotension accompanied by tachycardia.
c	**True**	Hypertensive patients demonstrate greater sympathetic activity in response to stress than normal individuals.
d	**True**	Tachyarrhythmias produced by laryngoscopy and intubation may be attenuated by pretreatment with beta-blockers.
e	**True**	Hypoxia causes tachycardia initially and subsequently may lead to bradycardia.

(Ch. 25, A & S)

a	**True**	It supplies all the intrinsic muscles of the hand apart from the lateral two lumbricals and the muscles of the thenar eminence.
b	**False**	See **a** above.
c	**False**	
d	**True**	This is employed in the use of electrical nerve stimulators to provide an evoked muscle response.
e	**False**	Cutaneous sensation to the medial one-and-a-half fingers is subserved by the ulnar nerve.

(Ch. 9, A & S)

a	**False**	Thiopentone has anticonvulsant properties.
b	**False**	Diazepam has anticonvulsant properties.
c	**True**	Substitution of a methyl group in the nucleus confers convulsive activity. The use of methohexitone in children with a history of epilepsy is contraindicated.
d	**True**	There is increased EEG spike activity during anaesthesia with enflurane. It is usually contraindicated in epileptics *(Ch. 8, A & S)*.
e	**False**	Spontaneous movements with suxamethonium are caused by fasciculations.

57 Hypothyroidism is associated with

a brisk ankle jerk.

b hair loss.

c pericardial effusion.
d malar flush.
e systolic murmur at the left sternal edge.

58 A tourniquet applied during orthopaedic surgery

a should be applied after exsanguination of the limb using an Esmarch bandage.
b is inflated to a pressure 50 mmHg > systolic arterial pressure if applied to the lower limb.
c should be deflated after a maximum of 2 h.
d should be deflated gradually to limit the release of metabolites.
e is contraindicated in the presence of severe peripheral vascular disease.

59 DC defibrillation may be used to correct

a atrial fibrillation.
b AV dissociation.

c multifocal ventricular extrasystoles.

d ventricular fibrillation.
e asystole.

60 Non-depolarizing neuromuscular blockade

a can be reversed by edrophonium.

b is antagonized only partially if neostigmine is used without atropine.
c may be monitored successfully using a double-burst stimulus of 50 Hz.
d is antagonized adequately if, on train-of-four (TO4) stimulation, the ratio of the fourth to the first twitch is 0.3.
e is affected by temperature.

(Ch. 8, D)

a **False** The ankle reflex is usually slower in the presence of hypothyroidism.
b **True** This is a well recognized feature and occurs especially in the outer one-third of the eyebrow.
c **True**
d **True** This is well described in hypothyroidism.
e **False** Flow murmurs are associated with hyperthyroidism, not hypothyroidism.

(Ch. 26, A & S)

a **True** But simple elevation of the lower limbs may suffice, especially if bilateral tourniquets are applied.
b **False** 100 mmHg > systolic pressure is recommended for the lower limbs.
c **True** It is usual to try to limit this to 1.5 h.
d **False** This manoeuvre has little effect on release of metabolites.
e **True**

(Ch. 3, D)

a **True** This may require synchronized defibrillation.
b **False** AV dissociation with an idioventricular rhythm is usually an indication for electrical pacing.
c **False** Treatment usually employs a membrane-stabilizing agent such as lignocaine.
d **True** This is usually the only effective form of treatment.
e **False** Asystole does not respond to DC defibrillation. In cardiac arrest in the absence of an ECG diagnosis, DC defibrillation should be employed, as no further harm will come to the asystolic patient.

(Ch. 11, A & S)

a **True** Edrophonium, a short-acting anticholinesterase, is employed commonly for reversal of non-depolarizing neuromuscular blockade.
b **False** The reversal of neuromuscular blockade by neostigmine is independent of any effect of atropine.
c **True** A double burst of 50 Hz tetany provides a visually acceptable monitor.
d **False** Reversal is usually adequate if the TO4 ratio is greater than 0.7.
e **True** Decreased temperature enhances the action of non-depolarizing neuromuscular blockers.